THE MAX
GOLF
WORKOUT

THE MAX GOLF WORKOUT

A Proven Regimen to Improve Your Strength, Flexibility, Endurance, and Distance off the Tee

John Little

SKYHORSE PUBLISHING

Skyhorse Publishing books may be purchased in bulk at special discounts for sales promotion, corporate gifts, fund raising, or educational purposes. Special editions can also be created to specifications. For details, contact Special Sales Department, Skyhorse Publishing, 555 Eighth Avenue, Suite 903, New York, NY 10018 or info@skyhorsepublishing.com.

www.skyhorsepublishing.com

10 9 8 7 6 5 4 3 2 1

Library of Congress Cataloging-in-Publication Data

Little, John R., 1960–
    The max golf workout : a proven regimen to improve your strength, flexibility, endurance, and distance off the tee / by John Little.
        p. cm.
    ISBN 978-1-60239-228-1 (alk. paper)
    1. Golf—Training. 2. Physical fitness. I. Title.
    GV979.T68L58 2008
    613.7'11—dc22   2007051235

Printed in China

DEDICATION

This book is dedicated to my wife, Terri, and to our children, Riley, Taylor, Brandon, and Benjamin, who encouraged me in the research, experimentation, and development of this protocol. It is also dedicated to my late father, William T. Little, who first introduced me to the game of golf (alas, when I was too young to appreciate it) and to Sally and Gord Sisco, who reintroduced me to the game many decades later. And finally, this book is dedicated to those individuals who value reason and science in their training and do not follow the "herd" mentality that so dominates popular culture.

CONTENTS

FOREWORD

When I first walked through the doors of Nautilus North Strength and Fitness Centre in 2004, I was "green" by fitness industry standards to the whole concept of strength training. Although I had read many books on strength training and had played sports and trained with weights for years, I had no way of knowing that there was a "right" way and a "wrong" way of exercising—and that I (and most everyone else) had apparently been misled by the industry into thinking that there were only "different" ways. I worked with John Little from that year to the present and we agreed to test everything—every workout protocol, every recovery interval, every nutritional consideration that we had heard about. As a result, many concepts that were popular were found to be without foundation, and a new direction began to emerge.

We conducted studies on protocols to test training theories on large numbers of people to see what worked, to what degree it worked, and whether or not better results could be obtained. As someone who likes to golf, my interest in how to improve my game was always in the back of my mind. Many of the clients I train are also golfers and are hungry for knowledge on ways to improve their games as well. What taking part in all of these studies gave was an objective view of the data. Neither I nor my clients cared about the fitness industry, or what was the new hot trend. Instead, we wanted results—the quicker the better—and if that meant we didn't have to be in the gym three to four days a week, that was fine by us as we'd rather be out golfing anyway.

In the first year that I worked for John and Terri Little I personally supervised some 7,500 workouts and our facility oversaw some 25,000 workouts. Indeed, since we kept workout records on all of our clients there was already a considerable database of cause and effect relationships prior to setting out to conduct our more formal studies into the effects of exercise.

One of our first studies involved devising a means to determine an individual's optimal training frequency. For instance, when did the body produce a change in muscle mass and at what point would it begin to lose size after it had been produced? The results were astonishing. The first few days following the workout revealed to us that a trainee is not stronger, but weaker. Indeed, since recovery precedes growth, the data revealed that a trainee is not ready to work out again and would not make any meaningful progress for at least a week after a workout. We also discovered that, despite what the fitness industry has been saying for years, one did not lose what one had gained if one did not work out again within ninety-six hours. With help of the Bod Pod body composition testing machine, we were able to scientifically track what happens to the body in the two weeks after a high intensity workout—this was the first time that such a test had been performed.

Then we wanted to see how much fat could be lost in a ten-week period. Again, this had relevance to the game of golf as muscle is what contracts (not fat) and it is muscular contraction that moves the clubs. However, we had seen that the fitness industry belief was that you had to spend multiple hours over multiple days per week in order to lose body fat. Was this true? Or was there a better, simpler way? These were questions we wanted answers for when we conducted our second study. The answers to these questions will surprise you and are laid out in this book. The combined time of all ten workouts is less than what most personal trainers would have you go through in your first session. This study not only will change how people look at fat loss but it also spoke to how little training is actually required to accomplish it.

By reading this book and following the training guidelines you will become a stronger athlete, and a stronger athlete is a better athlete. Will it bring you up to the upper levels of the PGA? Probably not, but it will certainly allow you to better your own game and allow you to chase that little white ball much longer and to hit it a hell of a lot farther—without living your life in the gym.

—Cary Howe

Lead trainer, Nautilus North Strength & Fitness Centre
Bracebridge, Ontario

INTRODUCTION: TOWARDS A NEW PERSPECTIVE

To begin, it should be pointed out that this is not a golf book. It will not at any point speak of how to grip a club, how to position your feet, the arc of the swing, graphite clubs, or the "inner game" of golf. It is assumed that the reader already has some knowledge of these facets of the game, and presently is looking for a means of improving his overall strength and fitness levels so as to be able to improve upon his ability to play the game of golf more efficiently and with greater power.

However, this is not merely a compendium of workout routines. Instead, within these pages you will learn of a revolutionary new perspective on strength training. It is so revolutionary (at least compared to what is being typically served up as strength training for golfers) that you will need to open your mind to new facts and, surprising as this may sound, common sense. To help the reader cultivate the correct mindset for learning, I have reworked a short Zen parable.

A golfer once learned that a new training protocol had been developed that had produced fast and startling improvement in one's golf game. As the innovator of this protocol lived in semi-seclusion in a northern town, he decided he would make the trip to speak with him. The innovator received the golfer graciously and invited him out onto his deck on a beautiful summer day to answer his questions.

"Tell me about this system of yours," began the golfer. As the innovator began to explain, he was frequently interrupted by the golfer: "Oh, yes, in the gym where I work out, my personal trainer has me do something like that," and "it sounds interesting in theory but nobody I know trains that way." After several fruitless attempts to explain himself uninterrupted, the innovator finally suggested that they have a cup of coffee. The golfer agreed. The innovator went into his home and came out with a pot of coffee and two cups. He poured his own and then began to fill the golfer's cup. As the golfer continued to talk about the traditions and methods of the sports greatest champions, the innovator kept filling his cup until it began to overflow. "What are you doing?" asked the golfer incredulously. "Can't you see that the cup is full?" "Precisely," answered the innovator. "Like this cup, you are so full of your own preconceptions, opinions and traditions, that there is no more room in your mind for what I have to say. Unless you first empty your cup, how will you ever taste my cup of coffee?" The golfer got the point.

I would ask that you, like the golfer, first "empty your cup" of all preconceived notions, opinions, and traditions on the subject of how to train for the game of golf so that you will have room—intellectually—for what I am about to relate.

Anatomists tell us that more than four hundred muscles are responsible for allowing us to go about our daily activities. It's also common knowledge that if we don't make an effort to use them to 100 percent of their energy potential, they'll slowly wither away with the passage of time. Ironically, while all of us possess the same number of muscles, not all of us possess the same number of muscle fibers in each of our muscle groups. This explains why few of us can ever develop our muscles (not that many of us wish to) to the same size as champion bodybuilders. Let it be understood that the champions of any sport—whether of yesteryear, today, and, for that matter, tomorrow possessed one quality that the vast majority of us do not—uncommon genetics. The strongest and most muscular among them had long muscle bellies, greater muscle fiber density, greater than average bone thickness, and higher than normal metabolisms. However, while only a certain portion of the population can develop a heavy musculature, everyone can improve their strength and the size of their muscles to a considerable degree, along with dramatically improving their performance in the game of golf—if they train intelligently, scientifically, and realistically.

For years golfers seeking to become stronger have known that weight training is the key. However, how to best employ weights in developing maximum strength and realizing one's full muscular potential has been a rather foggy area at best. This book is an attempt to bring some much-needed science into the arena of strength training with the specific goal of improving one's golf game. For decades there has been the belief that if one merely aped a particular golfing champion's training method, then one could dramatically improve one's game—a belief that has been found to be completely erroneous.

This is not to suggest that there isn't a way to improve such aspects of the game as the power of your drive, better control of your irons, and improved precision in putting. There is. However, it has little or nothing to do with such things as stretching, mental concentration exercises

It is time for golfers to take a fresh, unobstructed look at what their actual training requirements should be.

(for wishing will not make it so), or going to the gym three to four days a week to increase one's strength and muscular endurance. For too long, training for the game of golf has been left to the domain of uninformed personal trainers who seek nothing other than more billable hours, coaching folklore that has little scientific basis, and the subtle blandishments of the commercial interests that have infiltrated all sports and, indeed, all endeavors in which peak performance is a value. Science has been all but shut out because reality is often less alluring than fantasy.

Taking quite a different approach, this book is based upon three simple touchstones:

1. Research.
2. Research.
3. More research.

You will not find a word of advice within these pages that is not supported by scientific study. This book's conclusions and recommendations will, therefore, be refreshing to some (who enjoy new discoveries that can be validated empirically) and upsetting to others (particularly those with commercial ties to certain aspects of the fitness and golfing industry), while at the same time providing ample intellectual ammunition for those who sensed that something was amiss with the training advice they have been receiving, but had lacked the data necessary to counter such claims with any type of authority.

For over ten years I have helped golfers improve their strength and their game, but more importantly, I've continued to study human physiology and the role of strength training in helping people to optimize their potential and have continued to experiment and refine what I've learned. This book is the result.

The information contained within its pages will make you considerably stronger, fitter, and will dramatically improve your game of golf in the quickest, most efficient manner presently known by science. And it will further serve as a fact-checking guide for those who truly seek to obtain the most (or Max) from their bodies and from the game that they love so much.

—**John Little**

PART ONE:

THE DATA

1
WHERE ARE ALL THE TIGERS?

Genetics is the cardinal factor in creating an exceptional athlete.

The crowd is hushed as Tiger Woods makes his way to the tee. His swing is a picture of lithe beauty as the club arcs backwards, pauses ever so slightly at the apex of the ascent, and then changes direction seamlessly, picking up speed during the downswing. The club head connects with the ball and it rockets off from the tee, rising up seemingly into the clouds. The crowd loses sight of it until it drops down some 300 yards from where he is standing; dead center in the middle of the fairway. Another perfect drive by Tiger.

A short time later, Tiger chips onto the green from a distance of sixty feet. The ball overshoots the flag, and drops onto the green some ten feet away—but then seems to defy the laws of physics as it suddenly reverses gear and begins to roll backwards towards the cup. In what appears to be slow motion, the ball gradually zeroes in on the hole and, after an agonizing pause, drops into the cup. Tiger racks up another birdie.

"Wow!" an excited member in the crowd asks of no one in particular. "How did he do that?" Another member asks the question that most in the audience that day are only thinking: "What does it take for a person to be able to play at this level?" The answer to both questions is: ideal genetics.

Think of the greatest golfers—I mean the absolute top tier—of the past fifty years. Only a handful of names come to mind. Why? All of the golfers over the past fifty years trained for the game in exactly the same way that the greatest champions of their respective eras trained. They all worked on their swings and they relaxed. They kept their heads down and looked at the ball, they went out and bought new balls and clubs, they paid attention to the "inner game" of golf, and more recently, they have started to incorporate some form of weight training into their lives to "play more like Tiger does." So, if the majority of golfers today are all training more like Tiger does, the question remains: why aren't there more golfers like Tiger Woods walking around the local golf courses? And the answer, again, is genetics.

The fact is that somebody in Tiger Woods' family tree had spectacular hand-eye coordination, an uncanny ability to relax and focus under intense pressure, and the correct bone structure, muscle structure, and metabolic machinery to excel at the game of golf. All of these attributes were inherited by Tiger in just the right proportion which, when coupled with his almost daily neural/muscular practicing of the shots required within the game itself, allowed these traits to come to the fore and saw him blossom so spectacularly in the game of golf. This is why Tiger was on the Mike Douglas TV show at the age of two demonstrating his phenomenal aptitude for the game of golf, while you and I were refining our finger painting skills. A similar situation existed in John Daly's family tree; someone passed down the genetic factors necessary for him to be one of the greatest long ball hitters in the history of the game. (It certainly wasn't any training method he employed, since, by his own admission, he doesn't train at all!) Unless you, likewise, had ancestors that passed along such similar genetic traits, then you can adopt whatever aspect of your favorite golfer's program you want—but it simply won't make any difference; you'll never have the experience of getting sized for that Masters jacket.

You think I might be overstating the role of genetics in developing a champion? Well, consider that if you were to take a cross-section of 100,000 people, there might be 20 that possess the genetics necessary to become champions at the game of golf. Of those twenty, ten might be interested enough to take up the game, and of those ten, there might be one who would be intelligent enough to train and diet properly to fulfill his genetic potential for championship status. So the odds are 100,000-to-1 against you becoming a champion golfer. And this is why we see so few "Tigers" out on the fairways these days.

Just how big a role do genetics play in one's response to training? In a study that was conducted by M. C. Thibault and published in *Human Heredity* ("Inheritance of human muscle enzyme adaptation to isokinetic strength training." 36 (6):341–7, 1986), five sets of identical twins took part in a ten-week strength training program. The biochemical markers of strength were monitored during this time. At the conclusion of the study a wide range of response was noted between different twin sets, but the responses of the identical twin sets were, as you might have guessed, identical.

However, genetic potential—particularly for a game such as golf—is not nearly as tangible an aspect of an individual's physiology as other more measurable aspects, such as muscle length and thickness and bone structure. These are easily spotted in sports such as football, wherein the better linebackers display long torsos, short legs, wide hips, narrow shoulders and long arms, and top sprinters display short torsos, narrow hips, long legs, and a favorable ratio of the lower to the upper leg.

In golf, many of the factors that go into producing a champion are far less tangible, such as superior neuromuscular coordination, resulting in many groups of muscle fibers (motor units) contributing just the right amount of force at just the right time to result in powerful accurate drives, precision chips, and geometrically perfect putts. However, lest we forget, it is muscle in motion that that brings all of these factors together.

Genetic potential for excelling in the game of golf is not as easy to identify as it is in other sports.

2

A STRONGER GOLFER IS A BETTER GOLFER

Muscles are the engines that empower every facet of the golfer's game.

While science has known of the positive connection between strength and athletics for decades, there are still many amateur (and even a few professional) golfers who are of the opinion that strength is not an important component of the game of golf, or doubt that it even factors into the mechanics of a powerful golf swing. To be sure, these same individuals will expound eloquently on the importance of the "science" behind lighter clubs, the "physics" underlying a perfect swing technique, and the esoteric aspects of visualization and concentration, and as these are the individuals who tend to have media microphones thrust in front of them whenever they speak, it is only natural that these aspects of golf have received inordinate attention and thus have influenced the thinking of many golfers.

And while I'm not debating the significance of these elements, I believe the paradigm needs to be adjusted to reflect the reality of muscular strength not only in the generating of club head speed, but in all facets of the game.

This "anti-muscle" attitude is a throwback to the ancient belief that proper strength training will somehow make a person "muscle bound" and unable to move with freedom and fluidity. However, this attitude (as lawyers like to say) is groundless and without merit.

There are many within the golf industry that view muscle building as the "weak sister" of exercise. Building endurance, or greater stamina, is generally viewed as something separate from strength (which it is not). Flexibility is also viewed as something divorced from strength (which, again, it is not), the belief being that only certain twists, turns and pulls performed without resistance can optimize such things as our degree of trunk rotation and the degree of follow through with our drivers and irons.

It is the position of science, however, that muscle building is *the* most important factor in physical fitness and without it, the other two factors not only cannot be improved, but would not even exist. Every time you move, whether it be raising an eyebrow or taking a step, it is muscular action that is responsible. It is muscle that moves the limbs through their full range of motion (as in flexibility) and causes the heart (which is itself a muscle) to beat faster (as in endurance and cardiovascular efficiency). Tony Robbins, the internationally acclaimed peak performance coach, recently wrote in his introduction to my book *Max Contraction Training* that

> You can make all kinds of changes to your emotions, your relationships, but if you're physically unable to follow through on your decisions, it's all for naught. Unfortunately, one thing that I have learned, after more than a quarter of a century working with 3 million people from 80 different countries, is that most people don't truly realize how interconnected physical fitness—including strength training—is to fulfilling your potential at the highest level.

Let us, for the moment, divest the term "muscle" of its popular bodybuilding magazine and weightlifting connotations. It remains the *sine qua non* of human effectiveness on whatever plane of existence you may choose to evaluate our species. Muscle has built all the roads, cities, and machines in the world, written all the books, spoken all the words and, in fact, as Professor G. Stanley Hall wrote over 100 years ago:

> Muscles have, in fact, done everything that man has accomplished with matter. If they are underdeveloped, or grow relaxed and flabby, the dreadful chasm between good intentions and their execution is liable to appear and widen. Character might be in a sense defined as a plexus of motor habits. . . . The muscles are by weight about 43 percent of the average adult male human body. They expend a large portion of all the kinetic energy of the adult body. . . . The cortical centers for the voluntary muscles extend over most of the lateral psychic zones of the brain, so that their culture (the culture of muscles) is brain building. In a sense they are the organs of digestions. They are in a most intimate and peculiar sense the organs of the will.

Aware of the importance of muscle in human activity, virtually all of the better fitness centers today provide strength or resistance training equipment for their clients, along with advice on how to best strengthen your body. But whether or not you choose to join a fitness center or prefer to train at home with a home gym set up, it is vitally important to your total health and fitness that you engage in *some* form of muscle strengthening exercise.

So many of us rust out rather than wear out owing to a purpose-ful neglect of our muscles. Even those who exercise (particularly on their own) often fall far short of their full potential by neglect of proper muscle training. Many believe that they simply don't have the time for such training. After all, strength training requires at least several hours a week and a major lifestyle change, right? Wrong. Scientific research (including my own over the past two decades) has revealed that mus-cle size and strength—and even dramatic increases in cardiovascular

Research has clearly established that stronger muscles dramatically improve a golfer's performance.

conditioning and flexibility can be accomplished with as little as one training session per week that lasts between two and fifteen minutes. And the good news is that as you get stronger, even *less* training is required to continue to improve your level of strength fitness.

Increased muscular strength, then, will not only serve to improve your game of golf, but also your overall levels of health and fitness. With regard to golf, as the golf clubs don't move by themselves, it should be obvious that muscles are the engines that power every drive, chip, and putt. It is a rare golfer, indeed, who has the musculature of a gymnast or a ballet dancer, and yet these athletes are the models of grace and fluidity of movement. It is odd that some golfers (John Daly comes to mind) have allowed themselves to believe that training to add five pounds of extra muscle to their bodies isn't worth the effort, yet never ask how five pounds of extra fat will limit their movement—which it will.

3

A REVOUTIONARY STUDY—AND ITS IMPLICATIONS

A strength training study conducted in Boise, Idaho, over 10 years ago saw golfers improve their average off the tee distance by 15 yards.

Despite all of the press in recent years devoted to the "inner game" of golf and technique issues such as how to grip the club, it is doubtful that golfers who have been golfing for many years could merely adjust their grip or mental focus and see a twenty- or thirty-yard increase in their average drive, along with a boost in overall energy and physical power. However, if you gain muscle mass and strength, the geometry of your swing will improve, not decline. This was established during a study that I oversaw in Boise, Idaho, in 1997 that produced the following documented results:

- A thirty-one-yard increase in the distance of one subject's average drive distance.
- An increase of nearly fifteen yards for the average subject of the study.
- An average increase in overall body strength of 84 percent.
- An increase in stamina, better mental focus, balance, and superior athletic performance.

And all of the golfers who participated in this study achieved the above as a result of 6.6 workouts taking an average of just 2.2 minutes of actual exercise, or 14.5 minutes of total exercise time performed over a period of six weeks. Incidentally, there were four women who took part in the study—and they actually outpaced the four men in overall strength gains; the men achieved a 73 percent gain in strength (on average) while the women achieved a 95 percent gain. In case you were wondering how the muscle groups of the whole body could be thoroughly taxed by so little training time, here is the strength increase breakdown per muscle group:

- Chest +58%
- Back +60%
- Shoulders +57%
- Frontal thighs +86%
- Rear thighs +78%
- Abdominals +170%
- Lower Back +58%
- Calves +51%

- Triceps +133%
- Biceps +72%
- Forearm (flexors) +87%
- Forearm (extensors) +93%

* Overall Average Strength Gain +84%

And in case you are wondering, the subjects performed no stretching whatsoever. They did not ride an exercise bicycle or walk on a treadmill, and they did not roll around on big balls during their exercises. They also did not meditate or take acupuncture treatments or wear "ionized" bracelets, and no new "ultra light" clubs or radical new driving techniques were employed to obtain any of the above results. Moreover, this study was performed over a decade ago—and I've learned a lot more about the science underlying this process, and have refined it considerably since then.

Not only will your drives improve with proper strength training, but so will your short iron game.

Such dramatic results, along with the brevity of the training program that produced them are absolutely staggering (at least when contrasted with conventional workouts). However, the protocol and the results are firmly grounded in the sciences of physics and biology. Given that most golfers strength train these days, but few have achieved comparable results, there is something about this approach that bears serious consideration. Not only are the results substantially greater than conventional methods, but the time savings (thus giving the golfer more time to perfect his or her swing or engage in other life issues) represent a huge reprieve in one's weekly schedule.

The 1997 study cited above involved eight golfers, aged eighteen to fifty-eight. These men and women were given extremely short exercise routines consisting of only six exercises in which a weight was held motionless (instead of being pumped up and down) for a period of only ten to twenty seconds. After a mere six weeks, wherein each subject trained an average of once per week, the subjects had gained over fourteen yards on their average driving distance, were able to play more holes for longer periods of time without becoming fatigued, and also substantially shaped up their bodies—gaining muscle and losing body fat at the same time. What has made these results the talk of the golfing world (the study was reviewed in *Golf* magazine) is the fact that each workout took only two minutes to complete. In addition, the subjects in this study also reported improvements in their short-iron game, their stamina, their balance, and their confidence. The facts became clear: strength has the same importance as any other single factor in golfing and more importance than many other comparatively trivial issues that have received more attention over the years.

For years strength has been maligned or dismissed as being, at best, an unimportant consideration in improving the golfer's game. As a result of the data from this experiment, along with the fact that more and more professional and amateur golfers are now using strength training to augment their game (Tiger Woods is perhaps the most visible of this new breed of golfer), we now know that proper strength training is an absolutely critical factor in improving not only the golfer's overall levels of health and fitness, but in dramatically improving his or her game as well. This said, too much of a good thing can hurt your game and strength training is no exception, which is why the work-outs I advocate—and achieved such great success with—are very brief and performed very infrequently. Overtraining caused by the belief that "more is better" is worse than not engaging in strength training at all. It should be obvious, however, that golf is a muscular game; it requires muscles to swing your club, pivot your feet, rotate your hips, and arc your swing. In fact, if you are anything less than as strong as you can be, then you will be operating, by definition, at a sub-maximal standard.

When a golfer wishes to add more distance or power to his game, the answer lies in increasing the strength of the muscles he must utilize. However, for years this aspect of conditioning has all but been ignored in favor of less tangible factors. Now, however, compelling evidence is on hand to support the contention that a "stronger golfer is indeed

Golf is a muscular game.

a better golfer," and the good news is that it takes almost no time to become a stronger golfer.

As touched upon earlier, I know something about the particular study cited above, as I was the one who designed the training program that was employed during it, and recorded the measurements of the subjects' drive distances. However, in the years since that study was conducted, more data have been amassed to support the conclusion that infrequent workouts are most beneficial and that a particular protocol (or method of training) exists that will allow anybody to reach the upper limits of their genetic potential for strength in record time. In other words, there is a better way to become stronger, faster, than was employed during the course of the first study, and this constitutes a far more powerful technology for allowing you to become a much stronger, and much better, golfer.

4

A SECOND REVOLUTIONARY STUDY

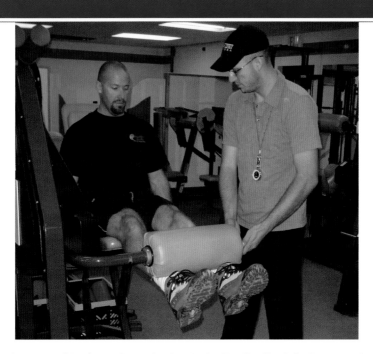

Trainer Cary Howe (right) was the lead trainer in the Nautilus North Study, overseeing each workout, recording the data, and assisting with the body composition testing.

When flipping through the pages of a golf book or magazine, there are usually a fair number of pages devoted to fitness and conditioning. None indicate when improvements will be produced from such efforts; rather the reader is told in a biblical commandment style that "Thou shalt stretch," or "Thou shalt lift weights to become stronger." Gains from following such directives, if mentioned at all, are expected to come sooner or later (and usually later), if the reader just employs these methods and keeps with the program long enough. However, gains from exercise shouldn't be a hit or miss affair. Proper training and its results are a simple matter of stimulus-response, and consequently the response (i.e., the result) should not be an unpredictable irregular phenomenon, but should (if properly applied) follow as soon as one's physiology allows.

Most golfers looking to gain strength typically lose sight of the fact that the models they are looking at in the pages of those magazines and books have been selected to model exercises solely because they are—from a physique perspective—among the genetically blessed; i.e., they have long muscle bellies and, more particularly, many more fibers packed into a given muscle than the vast majority of us. Consequently, when the physique model doubles the strength (and hence the effective cross section) of his muscles, they get much, much bigger than the average individual's whose genetics are not as strong. A champion bodybuilder, for instance, who has four times the muscle fiber density in his biceps than another individual, will, assuming both are training with sufficient intensity to double their mass, always have a muscle that is four times bigger than the average trainee's. With this in mind, the golfer must develop a more realistic perspective on what he might accomplish in terms of muscle mass increase through productive training. If one were to ask the model how he developed his muscles, the answer may be that he didn't do much of anything (remember the genetics component?). Similarly, if you ask a great golfer how he trains, his answer may yield you no benefit whatsoever (genetics again).

Many years ago, the late Arthur Jones (the founder of both Nautilus Sports/Medical Industries and the MedX Corporation) made the statement, "If you want to learn how to train a race horse, you don't ask the race horse." There is considerable merit in this statement as it has direct application to those who seek the advice of a champion in any sport, as genetic endowment is the prime determinant of athletic success, as well as an individual's response to exercise—of any stripe. This is not to suggest that features such as muscle size, shape, definition, flexibility, and endurance cannot be modified or enhanced to some degree by training, but even then, the influence and ultimate result will fall into a small range of degrees that are likewise genetically mediated.

As soon as any individual reaches a muscular size and strength level that his genetic predisposition has deemed to be adequate for his or her physiology, progress slows down dramatically or ceases altogether. At this point, simply doing "more" exercise, or switching routines does nothing to alter this fact of biology. Muscle growth, it should be pointed out, is a defensive reaction of the body to the stress of intense muscular contraction. If you can make your muscles contract twelve times (i.e., perform twelve repetitions) against a given load or resistance and you decide to arbitrarily terminate your set at eight repetitions, then your body has no reason to grow any bigger or stronger, because as far as it's concerned, it still has four reps in its gas tank—which you never came close to utilizing. This is why intense training, where one second more of muscular contraction simply isn't possible, is an absolute requirement for inducing muscle growth stimulation. Even if you did two, three, or ten more sub-maximal effort sets, you would only be re-stimulating the same fibers (and slow twitch ones at that; i.e., those with the lowest capacity to increase in strength and size), not involving (and thus stimulating) more fibers.

With this in mind, it stands to reason (and physiologists have proven this) that the sole stimulus to increased levels of size and strength is increased intensity of effort. The greater the intensity, the greater the growth stimulation. However, as intensity and volume (duration) exist in an inverse ratio to each other, it also is a matter of physiological fact that the harder or more intensely you do anything, the briefer must be the amount of time you can spend doing it. In other words, you can train hard with high intensity and brief duration or you can train easy with low intensity for long periods—but you can't train hard for long periods.

While the link between strength and golf has been clearly established, certain questions remain about what type of training will produce the fastest (maximum) results, how frequently one needs to expose oneself to the training stimulus for optimum results and how quickly one must wait to see discernible improvement in one's lean body mass composition. These were the issues I sought to answer with a study conducted at Nautilus North Strength & Fitness Centre in Bracebridge, Ontario, Canada.

It stood to reason that knowing precisely how soon a gain in muscle mass showed up after a workout had been performed would provide a trainee with the exact knowledge of how often he or she *should* train for optimal results. If, for instance, a gain in mass took two weeks to be produced, then what would be the point of training more than once every two weeks? All such extra training would succeed in doing is postponing

Nautilus North Strength & Fitness Centre in Bracebridge, Ontario (Canada), is one of the leading fitness research centers in North America.

or preempting the growth production process. If, however, the gains showed up in twenty-four hours, then waiting two weeks could possibly delay the gains to be had from proper strength training.

In addition, if such answers could be found, then an optimal training frequency could be determined from day one of a golfer's training career, resulting in the golfer doing everything possible to maximize each of his trips to the gym and every workout he performed. And as the golfer grew stronger and moved heavier weights in his workouts, he would not be required to train as often, for it only stands to reason that the energy required for his muscles to move those heavier weights would also be greater than the energy required for him to move lighter weights, and, consequently, it would take longer to replenish a greater energy deficit than it would to replenish a deficit of lesser magnitude (i.e., lifting 100 pounds for ten repetitions does not require as much energy as lifting 400 pounds for ten repetitions). In addition, periodic adjustments could also be made at future times to determine when the training frequency would need to be modified for both the intermediate and advanced level trainee by a similar process of experimentation to determine (again) their optimal training frequency.

The entire presently "gray" area of how often a golfer needed to train could suddenly be put into very black and white terms for each individual. This thought of breaking new ground is what served as my motivation in conducting this study.

The Nautilus North Study

Presently there are so many approaches and methods of training, it is almost impossible for someone of an experimental mindset to have a control group, as there's no way that a group of subjects will not know that they are not lifting weights. For this reason, I did not have a control group for this study. The control group would be anyone who doesn't lift weights and doesn't get stronger. After all, it is safe to assume that if people don't strength train, they won't (after puberty at least) grow stronger and bigger muscles.

And then came the decision as to what type of workout the subjects should do during the study. As our subjects were not beginners (where any type of training might produce results), we opted for advanced high intensity protocols that will be discussed shortly. The training stimulus had to be intense enough that there would be a high probability that muscle growth would be stimulated. And once stimulated, it should be produced if the body was given enough time to produce it. My main focus was centered on the questions of "when" the growth would be produced and "how much" of it would be produced. As each workout should produce a positive adaptation, the job of our technicians was then to test when this adaptation manifested.

As training ought to be purposefully directed, I went to what science had to say about how to strengthen a muscle and what type of contraction was necessary to do so, and then obtained a group of subjects who were willing to submit to sophisticated body composition testing on a

The data from the Nautilus North Study was first broken to the international public by *Ironman* magazine in 1995.

daily basis over a period of fourteen days in order to determine when the gains (however great or miniscule) would show up, thus revealing the absolute soonest one could train again without disrupting the process of recovery and growth.

With respect to how many such sets are required to produce optimal size and strength increases, the *Journal of Exercise Physiology* (online) published a most enlightening article in which, after an extensive review of all of the peer-reviewed scientific literature regarding training protocols, they concluded that one set taken to a point where an additional repetition was not possible was all that was required for building muscle size and strength in subjects with normal (i.e., non-drug enhanced) physiology.

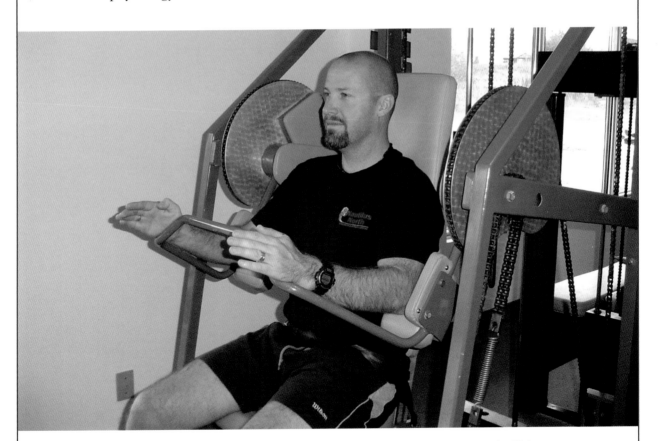

Each workout should produce a positive adaptation—if it's performed properly and sufficient time is allowed for recovery.

On a personal note, at Nautilus North Strength & Fitness Centre, which is owned and operated by my wife Terri and me, we have found by personally supervising over 42,000 workouts on a one-on-one basis that, unless an individual is grossly underweight, it is very difficult to put more muscle on him. Not impossible, only difficult. More difficult in that it requires an intensely focused effort on the part of the average trainee, and "average trainees," as a group, are not typically inclined to invest intense effort into their workouts unless they have a personal trainer who not only has a record of what they did in their previous workout (in terms of weight and repetitions) but is also able to motivate them to work out at their highest possible level. Such training is productive but not a lot of fun, with the result that most prefer to train at a modest level of intensity, two to three times per week, and precisely because their intensity is low, they don't need longer recovery periods as their weights (and correspondingly their strength levels) don't usually go up too much after their first month of training, and the stresses on the body likewise are capped. Their progress, in other words, ceases and they continue going to the gym because they believe it's "good" for them in some nebulous way or because it has become a ritual of sorts in their lives. I decided to check what would happen with clients who are very motivated to become stronger and leaner for their activities of work, sports (baseball, football, golf, and hockey), and other day-to-day existence issues. In other words, these individuals were motivated to become as strong and fit as they possibly could, thus fulfilling their genetic potential for muscular strength and size. The individuals who took part in this study were not grossly underweight or overweight, nor were they under-conditioned, being instead young-to-middle-aged-men, several of whom were fresh out of college where some ran and were coached in track and field. They were fit, quite muscular, and already very strong, but I wanted to see when the muscular gain that they stimulated from their workouts would be produced over the course of a two-week period. As the subjects would not be regaining previously held muscle mass and were already fairly well developed (regarding their individual genetic potentials for mass and strength), any gains—if they were genuine lean tissue (i.e., real muscle)—would be noteworthy and of significance to those interested in building muscle.

First, however, we needed a reliable means by which to track and assess body composition.

Enter the Body Comp Weight Analysis Center

It is very difficult for athletes and members of the general public to accurately test body composition. While it's true that there is no

All subjects in the Nautilus North Study had their body composition tested at Body Comp, a company that employs state-of-the-art technology.

shortage of body composition testing methods available, it is also true that not all of them are accurate (some can be in error by upwards of 30 percent). Moreover, without an accurate and repeatable means of assessing body composition, you are a rudderless ship. How do you know if your training and/or diet are producing any muscle gain at all? An individual can easily gain ten pounds over the course of a month—but ten pounds of what? Water? Fat? Muscle? Fat and muscle? A body-weight scale can't determine the difference, as its sole function is to record gross bodyweight—not determine its composition. The same applies to using a tape measure (another typical fitness industry means of assessing progress); putting two inches on your arm means nothing if those two inches are fatty tissue—and a tape measure, like a body-weight scale, merely measures volume—not the composition of that volume. To make any sort of meaningful measurement relevant to determining the productivity or relative lack thereof of a given training approach, the composition of the weight and volume gained has to be accurately assessed. You need to know, in other words, that the weight you gained from training this month was as a result of an increase in the lean composition of your body rather than fat. And conversely, if you are seeking to lose fat, you need to have a reliable means by which to know if the weight you lost was fat, water, lean tissue, or a combination of all three.

Options

A Dual Energy X-Ray Absorptiometry (DEXA) machine is good for this purpose, even being sophisticated enough to measure individual limbs for compositional components down to the gram—however, DEXA uses radiation and, even though it is present in small amounts, who wants to be exposed to radiation in any form or magnitude for repeated sessions? To consistently and accurately measure body composition, repeated testing is required over a short span of time—daily in our study—in order to determine when the gains actually are produced and what the immediate effects of a proper muscle building workout are on one's muscle physiology. DEXA, while valuable for bone densitometry, which is not required to be performed so frequently, simply posed more risk than value for our purposes. Underwater weighing

It resembles the inside of a space ship, but the Bod Pod capsule is probably the most accurate means of determining body composition on a regular basis.

(hydrostatic) is excellent and very accurate. And while hydrostatic weighing was the gold standard of body composition twenty years ago, there have been advances in composition assessment methods since that time, most notably in the areas of practicality and convenience. After all, who wanted to be dunked up to ten times for thirty seconds in an underwater tank? Moreover, I wasn't interested in having my subjects drive the hour and a half to Toronto and waiting for appointments in university physiology labs to use them. Moreover, most universities aren't interested, nor do they encourage, members of the general public to use their facilities—and certainly not as frequently as our testing required.

Bioelectric Impedance Analysis seemed promising but problems appeared with regard to both accuracy and repeatability with this technology; one client, a medical doctor in town, has a niece who is morbidly obese. He, by contrast, is a fitness freak; performing not only strength training but also competing in cross-country ski events. He is so defined that you can see virtually every muscle on his body. However, when both he and his niece tested themselves on a Bioelectrical Impedance machine, they both tested at 36 percent! Evidently, many of these machines only measure the composition of the limb or limbs in contact with their apparatus; as the current lacks strength to measure all aspects of the body. And who would want a super-charged electrical current running through their bodies, which would be required to increase the accuracy rate?

Calipers were another option, but as body fat is stored all over the body and not just in the three to four areas tested, there is no way that overall body fat can be accurately measured with such limited measurements (similarly, when body fat is lost, it comes off in a random order from all over the body and not just from the sites that the tests are conducted at). In addition, as calipers only measure subcutaneous fat deposits, their results would tell us nothing about visceral fat (or internal fat), which is the fat that typically builds up to cause serious health problems.

Moreover, of all the methods listed above, calipers have been shown to have the highest error percentage, typically the result of individuals storing fat often in different areas than those being measured at the sites the calipers target.

The only valid scientific method that I found that was ideal for the type of consistent, frequent, repeatable, and reliable whole body composition testing was that offered by Body Comp Weight Analysis Centre. They utilize the same principle of displacement that hydrostatic weighing employs, but rather than displacing water, their machine (a "Bod Pod" capsule) measures air displacement. The testing procedure is quick (under five minutes) and accurate to a plus-minus of 2 percent, which puts it on a par in terms of accuracy with hydrostatic weighing and, shy of an autopsy, is as accurate a measurement as science presently permits. Moreover, although this technology is used in universities, hospitals, and other professional institutions, this is the only one we were aware of (at least at the time of this writing) in Canada that is open to the general public. Utilizing this revolutionary technology, we were able to test the subjects in the study and know—to 0.1 of a pound—whether or not the weight the individual trainee was gaining or losing was lean or fat and whether or not a particular training and recovery protocol stimulated and allowed for the production of lean tissue—and, even more impressively, we were able to determine exactly—to the day—when this gain or loss showed up.

The Stimulus

The workouts were engineered so as to target the major muscle masses of the body in order that the likelihood of stimulating more muscle into growth would be realized. The workout employed no more than five (low) to eleven (high) sets per workout. Each of these sets were taken either to a point of positive (isotonic) muscular failure, negative (eccentric-only) failure, static failure, or Infitonic failure. (Note: Infitonic is a term coined by my late friend and bodybuilding pioneer Mike Mentzer to describe a technique whereby a subject would perform a maximum single [or isotonic] lift concentrically, followed immediately by a maximum negative or eccentric lift. This constitutes one repetition. A ten-second rest-pause is then taken, which delayed or prevented the build up of metabolites such as lactic acid that can compromise a maximum intensity contraction from being performed. This sequence is then repeated for a maximum of five repetitions.)

After the stimulus or workout was applied, the subjects were instructed to do no additional resistance exercise and they simply went about their

day-to-day affairs for the next fourteen days. To obtain a "ground zero," all of the subjects were given body composition tests prior to the workout stimulus being applied. As I was checking solely for lean (muscle) tissue increases, the subjects were not instructed to either increase or reduce their daily caloric intake. I wanted the sole variable to be the training stimulus. As a reduction in calories could compromise the lean content of the body (as if calories are restricted too low, lean tissue is often sacrificed to make up the differential), we knew that if the subjects ate their usual calorie intake (which they did) they would not sacrifice muscle tissue. This wasn't a "weight gain" study which typically sees the subjects eating more and gaining predominantly fat tissue; this was a study the sole focus of which was to determine how long it took the benefit (a bigger muscle) derived from a workout to be produced, and how much of it would be produced.

The Results of the Two-Week Study

Name	Start Lean	Finish Lean	Day of Peak Lean	Day of Lowest Lean
C. Greenfield	165.9	166.6	Day 10 (169.8)	Day 5 (160.7)
D. Craig	120.9	121.6	Day 5 (123.7)	Day 10 (118.6)
D. Beaudry	138.2	138.7	Day 1 (143.1)	Day 9 (137.8)
C. Bell	140.6	142.3	Day 6 (143)	Never went below 140.6
J. Biggs	171.9	171.5	Day 1 (173.8)	Day 4 (169)
I. Heshka	173.1	172.2	Day 7 (175.2)	Day 8 (170)
C. Howe	137.9	138.9	Day 10 (139.4)	Day 7 (135.6)
J. Little	144.5	146	Day 11 (146.7)	Day 1 (142.8)
J. Ostertag	120.9	120.1	Day 5 (122.6)	Day 1 (120.1)
T. Peake	138.4	143.2	Day 6 (147.7)	Day 9 (137.7)
J. Williams	142.4	144.1	Day 9 (145.7)	Day 3 (140.9)

Subjects were placed in the Bod Pod capsule every day for 14 days after their workout and three separate body composition tests were made. Factors such as age, gender, predicted lung volume, height, and weight were entered into the computer. After the test was completed the data indicating the percentage and poundage of lean and fat were printed out and shared with the subject to determine his optimal frequency.

Lean Gain in Two Weeks (in Pounds) Over Starting Level of Lean

Name	Start Lean	Finish Lean	Day of Peak Lean	Day of Lowest Lean
C. Greenfield	165.9	166.6 (0.7)	Day 10 (3.9)	Day 5 (−5.2)
D. Craig	120.9	121.6 (0.7)	Day 5 (2.1)	Day 10 (−2.3)
D. Beaudry	138.2	138.7 (0.5)	Day 1 (4.9)	Day 9 (−0.4)
C. Bell	140.6	142.3 (1.7)	Day 6 (2.4)	No low read
J. Biggs	171.9	171.5 (−0.4)	Day 1 (1.9)	Day 4 (−2.9)
I. Heshka	173.1	172.2 (−0.9)	Day 7 (2.1)	Day 8 (−3.1)
C. Howe	137.9	138.9 (1)	Day 10 (1.5)	Day 7 (−2.3)
J. Little	144.5	146 (1.5)	Day 11 (2.2)	Day 1 (−1.7)
J. Ostertag	120.9	120.1 (−0.8)	Day 5 (1.7)	Day 1 (same as start)
T. Peake	138.4	143.2 (4.8)	Day 6 (9.3)	Day 9 (−0.8)
J. Williams	142.4	144.1 (1.7)	Day 9 (3.3)	Day 3 (−2.5)

The above numbers indicate not body weight, but lean weight. The actual weight of the subjects—as measured by a scale—was considerably higher than indicated above, but as I was only interested in lean (or muscular) bodyweight, that is the only reading I have presented. The most striking gain was recorded by T. Peake, who produced 9.3 pounds of muscle after a mere six and a half days, and was up 4.8 pounds of muscle after two full weeks of body composition testing (all of this from only one workout). Such a rate of increase, if it could be sustained (which is very unlikely) would have seen him gain 9.6 pounds of muscle per month (and, if it was capable of being sustained into the future, 115.2 pounds of muscle per year). As this would be an unprecedented rate of increase, it is more likely that his rate of gain would arrest at some point, although we can't know in advance precisely when or what this point would be. Moreover, given that muscle will continue to respond with increases in size and strength providing it receives both the stimulus for change and the time required to produce such change, one must grant that such a gain, while heretofore unprecedented, is nevertheless possible statistically.

More likely, we should look to the *average* gain experienced by the subjects as something more realistic and therefore attainable. In determining the averages, I have presented the actual gains/averages from all of the subjects in the study, followed by the actual gains/averages with the highs and lows factored out in order to determine a more likely average for those of more average genetics and recovery ability:

Averages of all study participants

Beginning Lean Mass:	144.97
Ending Lean Mass:	145.93
Gain in Lean Mass:	0.955
Peak Lean Mass:	148.23
Gain in Lean at Peak:	3.27
Day of Peak Gain:	6.5
Lowest Lean Before Peak:	143.77
Pre-Peak Loss of Lean:	1.20
Day of Pre-Peak Loss:	1.9
Overall Lowest Lean:	143.07
Overall Loss of Lean:	1.90
Day of Overall Lowest Lean:	5.18

Averages (after factoring out the highs and lows)

Beginning Lean Mass:	144.52
Ending Lean Mass:	145.88
Gain in Lean Mass:	0.733
Peak Lean Mass:	148.10
Gain in Lean at Peak:	2.80
Day of Peak Gain:	6.6
Lowest Lean Before Peak:	143.17
Pre-Peak Loss of Lean:	0.8
Day of Pre-Peak Loss:	1.5
Overall Lowest Lean:	142.80
Overall Loss of Lean:	1.74
Day of Overall Lowest Lean:	5.22

A New Observation: Muscular Suppression

You will note that a pattern to muscle growth is evident from the data: the lean composition of human muscle actually dipped or was suppressed after the stimulus/workout was applied, reaching a low at Day 5 (on average) and not coming up for several days afterwards. Evidently, muscle tissue is somewhat like a sponge; immediately after an intense workout it is, for want of a better term, *compressed*; its constituents, some of which we know (such as glycogen), are used up and not immediately replaced, with the result that the lean composition of the body can actually be reduced or go down by several pounds and stay this way for several days after a workout. But then, over time, the lean tissue fills back up again and, if the workout has been sufficiently intense enough to stimulate a compensatory build up of new tissue, it will grow back bigger than it was prior to the previous workout. In other words, the muscle growth process is not an entirely linear progression; the muscle content of the body first gets smaller, then proceeds to increase in its volume with periodic ebbs and flows throughout the process until it finally returns (recovers) to its pre-workout size and then gets a little bit bigger (overcompensates).

No Decompensation in Forty-Eight to Ninety-Six Hours

Whereas certain trainers and even exercise physiology professors have long advised athletes that decompensation (or loss of muscle tissue from disuse) occurs after forty-eight or ninety-six hours (which is the rationale underlying multiple training sessions per week), our study revealed no evidence of this. In fact, it often took in excess of seven days or 178 hours for the gains to even be produced. Knowing this, and the fact that the muscles must first recover before they can grow, we can infer that training before peak growth has taken place will only keep the muscle tissue suppressed and postpone the maximum production of new muscle. The average peak gain from the workout arrived almost a full seven days later, and a large portion of the peak gain produced by the body was held right up until testing ended on Day 14.

With this data, we can now make some predictions of rate of muscle gain based upon a continued growth pattern and the trainee hitting his targeted peak training day and also predictions of the rate of growth by those who train even as little as once every two weeks (so much for "not finding the time" to workout!). The predictions are indicated below:

Predictions

Training once every 6.6 days	Training once every 14 days
Base Value: 2.800	Base Value: 0.733
After 1 week: 2.970	After 1 week: 0.367
After 2 weeks: 5.393	After 2 weeks: 0.733
After 4 weeks (1 month): 11.879	After 4 weeks (1 month): 1.466
After 2 months (8 weeks): 23.758	After 2 months (8 weeks): 2.932
After 6 months (26 weeks): 77.21	After 6 months (26 weeks): 9.529
After 1 year (12 months): 154.424	After one year (12 months): 19.058

A practical application

Based on the data from this study, the average peak day was 6.5 days. If we drop the highs and the lows to get a better average, we see that the average extends out to 6.6 days. The average muscular suppression or dip day occurs at day 1.9 and continues for several days thereafter.

As there are those who lead very busy lives, often working long hours and having families to raise, the knowledge that tremendous gains in

Optimum Training Frequency

Cary Home Optimum Training Frequency

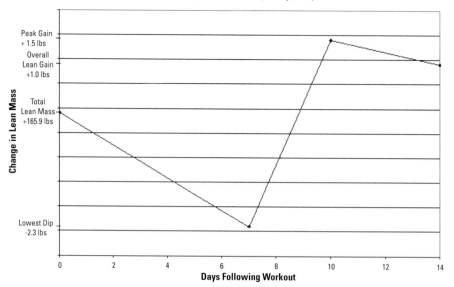

strength and muscle mass can be gained with as little as one workout every two weeks should be most emboldening. The average gain worked out to be 0.733, or just under three-quarters of a pound of muscle per two-week period and 5.93 pounds in two weeks (based upon the peak growth point). Such gains are considerable, as it will see the average trainee (with those of above average genetics gaining more, and those of below average genetics gaining less) gaining approximately nineteen and half pounds of solid muscle in one year. Moreover, this gain is achieved not by training every day, not by taking expensive supplements or drugs, not by drinking gallons of milk, but by eating normally and training but once every two weeks. You might have reason to be upset if you've been having your personal trainer work you out three or four days a week with the net result that your muscles are smaller and weaker.

If you didn't gain nineteen and a half pounds of muscle this past year, then paying attention to the "compression" or dip of lean tissue prior to the growth being produced is particularly noteworthy as it is a phenomenon that was observed in the vast majority of subjects and is, I suspect, applicable to the vast majority of trainees. Ignoring what

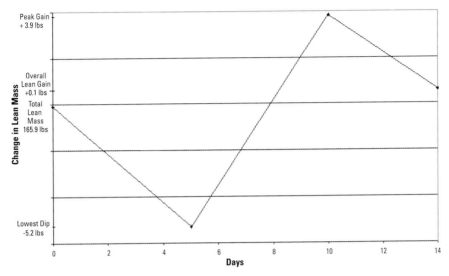

Chris Greenfield Optimal Training Frequency

would appear to be a biological law such as this could explain why many athletes fail to make the progress that they are capable of—and why training with weights several days each week is always a mistake.

Subject Cary Howe's Optimal Training Frequency

Subject Cary Howe's optimal training frequency occurs at Day 10. If he were to train on Day 6 (the average peak gain day for those on the study) he would actually be down, owing to muscular suppression, by 2.3 pounds. His optimal training frequency is once every ten days. If he waited until Day 14 he would lose one-third (or half a pound) of the lean tissue he stimulated.

Subject Chris Greenfield's Optimal Training Frequency

Subject Chris Greenfield's optimal training frequency is also longer than the "average," requiring ten days to elapse between workouts for peak adaptation to take place. Although he is tracking upwards by Day 6 (after five days of muscular suppression), his lean is well below his starting or pre-workout level. It is only on Day 8 that his lean is back to his pre-workout level, and Day 10 before it hits its peak. If he waits until Day 14 he will still be stronger and leaner (by three quarters of a pound) than he was prior to his previous workout, but well below what his peak level was on Day 10.

Such gains—between 0.733 and 2.97 pounds (depending upon average and peak gains) per week—of real muscle—produced in two weeks are very significant. Simple addition will reveal that if this rate of progress could be sustained, an individual would end up gaining as much as nineteen and a half pounds in one year by training once every two weeks.

It does not follow, however, that if one trained once a week that that he would end up gaining thirty-nine pounds (or twice the amount) of muscle in one year, given the mediating role of genetics in the muscle building equation. Most likely, the 19.5 pounds would be closer to the ceiling of one's potential (although, again, this will depend upon a given individual's genetic makeup), irrespective of whether one trained once a week or once every two weeks (with the once a week training, this potential might well be realized in a shorter period of time, say, six to eight months, rather than twelve). In either case, it would very likely see a given individual reach his full strength and muscular potential—whatever it may be—in one year or less. At the very least, these new data suggest that such is at least possible mathematically and to some degree possible biologically.

I would suspect that such gains, if and when they are forthcoming, would be almost solely dependent upon a given individual's genetic potential, which is something I cannot predict with infallible certainty in advance of the realization of such potential. If an individual reading this believes that he has better genetics than those of the subjects we trained in this study, it only stands to reason that the same protocol and frequency will produce even more impressive gains. After all, if a subject has more muscle fiber density, i.e., more muscle fibers per square inch of muscle, more fibers will be stimulated to grow bigger and stronger. And, if a less intense training approach, or a training approach that is too long (thus using up too much of an individual trainee's recovery ability), is coupled with insufficient recovery time, even a subject with superior genetics will be unable to realize his or her full strength and muscular potential.

PART TWO:

THE METHOD

5
UNDERSTANDING THE PROCESS

Proper exercise is a stimulus that acts upon the body. The body itself produces the response that exercise stimulates (such as an increase in muscle strength and size), and does so during the recovery period in between workouts.

In order to better understand what a scientific training program can do for you, it might help to understand something of the process that we are attempting to engage whenever we exercise. Exercise is nothing more than a stimulus that acts upon the body. That stimulus must cause a sufficient drain of the body's (or, more specifically, the muscles') energy system to cause the body to protect itself and its energy reserves against potential future assaults of like severity by making an adaptive response. This response takes place during a period of rest that follows the application of the stimulus.

Energy is the key word in this process. We are beings that have survived periods of starvation in our history because our bodies evolved the capability to conserve energy. This ability allowed us to hang in there during lean times for a few extra weeks until we reached a different location that yielded a greater food supply (energy). Failing this, the body also cultivated an ability to diminish the size of tissues (like muscle) that require a higher calorie (energy) expenditure from the body in order to be sustained. Consequently, our genetic programming, coming down to us as it has over eons, can be simply stated like this:

OUR BODIES LIKE	OUR BODIES HATE
High Energy In	Low Energy In
Low Energy Out	High Energy Out

If we were to graph the growth and decline of human strength and lean tissue from the moment we are born until the day that we die, it would form a perfect bell curve. It would appear, metabolically speaking, that the day we are born we are shot out of a cannon, and we ride that wave until we hit the apex of our lean (muscle) and strength, which happens to fall at the very peak of the bell curve (occurring at roughly age twenty-five), followed by a gradual tapering off until it declines to the same level as our starting point. Shadowing this curve (roughly above it) would be our genetic potential for increasing our size and strength, which we would realize—if we used our muscles to 100 percent of their momentary ability during our lifetime.

Some of us may participate in vigorous athletics between the ages of sixteen and twenty-six, which would see that graph bump up a little bit (or a lot, depending upon how much of our muscles' energy reserve was called upon for the activities we performed); in which case, that graph would move proportionally a little bit closer to our genetic potential for strength and size. However, most of us (including athletes) never use our muscles at a level anywhere near 100 percent of their capacities and, consequently, nature, being an economist at heart, begins at age twenty-six to make cost cuts for energy efficiency. If, for instance, we have a fourteen-inch arm but routinely use our arm muscles at an energy output that would only justify the size and strength of a twelve-inch arm, then our arm size will be reduced accordingly. And so it goes for each muscle group of the body.

By the time most of us reach the age of forty, we have lost a great deal of our muscle mass. The result is that our resting metabolic rate has

Our genetic programming is such that we will conserve energy whenever possible—such as taking a golf cart rather than walking the course.

slowed down considerably; the Kraft Dinner, pizza, and beer we lived on in college to no ill effect now seem to go directly to our midsections (or hips and thighs if you happen to be female) and activities that we used to take for granted now—should we decide to attempt them at all—leave us gasping for air and feeling like we've just climbed a very tall building with our cars on our backs. It is at age forty that most of us feel that we've "got to do *something* to get back in shape." So what do we do? We typically seek out the advice of a fitness professional—that is, someone who owns a gym. What we aren't expecting, however, is that the average fitness professional (and there are admittedly exceptions to this statement) is concerned about one thing only: turnover. That is the lifeblood of the fitness industry. The more people that will pay for a membership, the more money the individual gym owner can make and the longer he can stay in business. Toward that end, the market dictates what sells, and since getting people to work very hard and to exhaust the energy resources in their muscles is a very hard sell indeed, the fitness industry has compromised and has sold low intensity (low energy) activity as the prescription for the ailment of most people's loss of muscle and lowered metabolic rates. Given the genetic disposition of what our bodies like and dislike, the gym owners have opted for what is popular; i.e., selling the idea of going to the gym more frequently to exert small levels of energy is comfortable, and also satisfies the psychological wish of trainees to feel as though they are, in fact, doing "something" about their deteriorating physical condition. And while "something" they may be doing, it is not the required *something* that will turn that bell curve around and get them back to the level of lean that they enjoyed at age twenty-five. For this to take place requires the application of a very specific type of stimulus; i.e., one that gives the body a reason to rebuild previously held muscle—which, in turn, requires utilizing 100 percent of that muscle's energy reserves. As mentioned earlier, muscle growth, particularly new muscle growth, is a defensive reaction of the body to the stress of exercise, and the body must literally be forced to see the necessity of adding more strength and size. And as I ask the audiences at my seminars: "How do you force growth with mild exertion, light weights, and easy workouts?" And the answer is: You don't.

It takes hard training to build stronger muscles and, unfortunately, the fitness industry long ago sold us on the concept that exercise should be "fun" and leave you feeling "refreshed." While recreational activities can certainly do this, exercise—real exercise—does not. Exercise leaves you feeling literally "exhausted," because that is what you were training to accomplish; i.e., an exhaustion of the energy reserves within your muscles, and these reserves are not replenished for several days following the workout.

"What about working out at 10 percent of a muscle's capacity—and simply doing ten sets of an exercise? Wouldn't that net you out at 100 percent of your muscle's energy reserves?" No. The key words here are "10 percent." If you work out with 10 percent of the load that your muscles can contract against, or if you work out at 10 percent of what your muscles can do (in terms of repetitions) and then stop when it starts to feel uncomfortable, then you will have only used 10 percent. If you do this for nine more sets, you are still only operating within 10 percent of that muscle's capabilities and, consequently, there exists no stimulus to change anything at all about that muscle. To your body, that muscle is fine just the way it is because it still has a generous amount of energy in reserve (90 percent, to be exact), so what reason exists for it to enlarge the size of that muscle's "gas tank"? One set that utilizes 100 percent of your muscle's energy reserves, by contrast, is a huge stimulus for change, with the result that your body *will* change. Once you understand both your body's natural inclination not to exert energy and the fact that only by exerting 100 percent of a muscle's energy will you have provided sufficient stimulus to warrant change, you can begin to appreciate why "fun," "easy," "invigorating," and "social" are not terms to be associated with the activity of demanding (i.e., capable of producing significant positive change) exercise. And while your muscles might well be able to recover from a 10 percent effort sufficiently to be able to tolerate three to four weekly visits to the gym, you will not be stimulating your body to produce much (if any) change. And, conversely, if you exhaust your energy reserves to the degree necessary to stimulate change, you will not be able to recover from such an energy expenditure nearly so quickly. The greater the energy out, in other words, the longer it takes to put it back in.

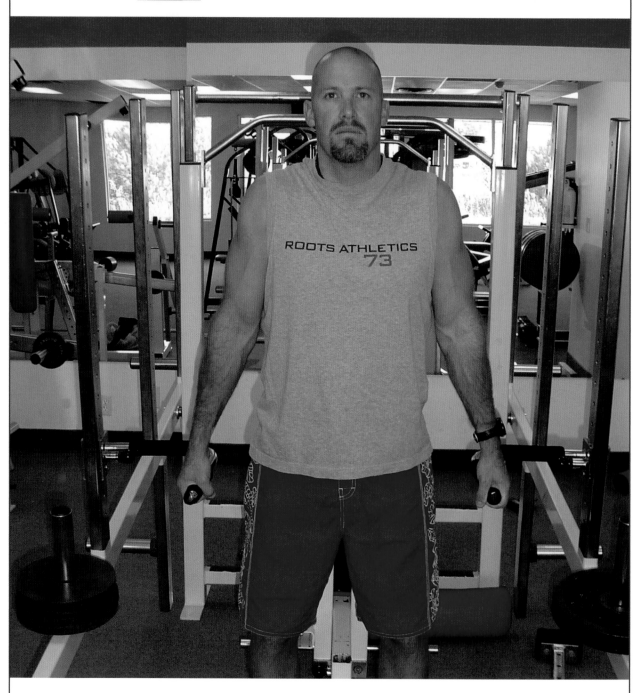

The body will not produce more muscle unless it absolutely has to—which is why easy
workouts with light weights simply won't cut it.

The process, put another way, is three-fold in nature:

- Stimulate (energy is drained from the muscle or muscles during the workout at a very high level).
- Recover (replenish the energy that was expended during the workout).
- Grow (adapt by enlarging the energy reserves within the muscle).

These last two phases of the process each require time and, as the Nautilus North study established, this time can take anywhere between 6.6 and 14 days (and perhaps longer, depending upon how profound the stimulus is in terms of exhausting the energy reserves in the muscle/s). I can tell you that we have personally supervised tens of thousands of

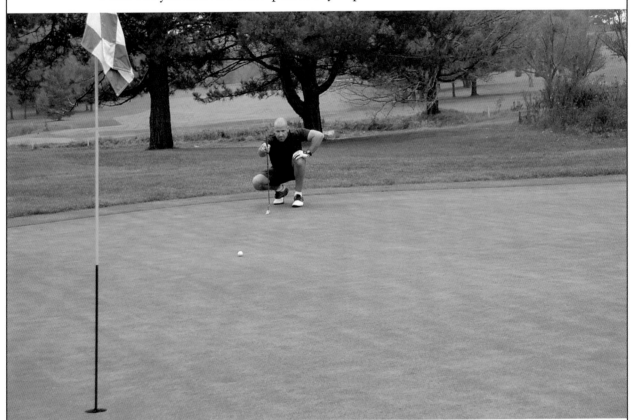

Don't be afraid to allow more recovery time in between your workouts. Remember, growth doesn't take place in the gym, it takes place while you are at rest (i.e., out of the gym).

workouts, using all sorts of training programs, over the past four years and invariably those who trained the most gained the least. The clients who are making the best progress at our fitness facility are training very intensely, very briefly and *very* infrequently. For now, this information should whet your appetite to train a little more intensely and to understand the necessity of allowing more recovery time to elapse between your workouts. After all, the growth you have stimulated in the gym is only produced when you are at rest; i.e., out of the gym, which, as we have seen, takes, in most instances, from seven to fourteen days (or longer).

6
THE MAX GOLF WORKOUT

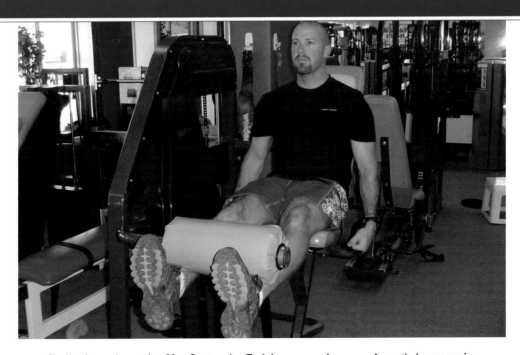

Studies have shown that Max Contraction Training can produce very dramatic increases in muscle strength and size.

One must perform those exercises with maximal or near maximal resistance to bring forth the greatest strength increments. The muscles will adapt only to the load placed upon them; a minimal overload will bring about minimal strength gain, whereas a maximal overload will bring about a maximal strength gain.

—Dr. David R. Lamb
Physiology of Exercise: Responses and Adaptations

The subject who gained the most rapidly in the Nautilus North study was Ontario resident Tim Peake. Peake's rate of progress, isolated from the rest of the group, was far above average. This most likely was a result of his genetic predisposition to build muscle mass. However, the fact that he trained on the Max Contraction protocol is also a factor. Let's look again at Tim's results in isolation from the rest of the group:

Tim Peake's Results After One Max Contraction Workout

Start Lean	Finish Lean	Day of Peak Lean	Day of Lowest Lean
138.4	143.2	Day 6 (147.7)	Day 9 (137.7)

Lean Gain in Two Weeks (in Pounds) Over Starting Level of Lean

Start Lean	Finish Lean	Day of Peak Lean	Day of Lowest Lean
138.4	143.2 (+4.8)	Day 6 (+9.3)	Day 9 (–0.8)

At the start of the study, Tim weighed 193.2 pounds. At the end of the study he weighed 192.7 pounds. If one were to go solely by gains on a bodyweight scale, one would conclude that Tim's Max Contraction workout produced a half-pound *loss*. However, since we utilized an ultra high tech body composition testing machine (air displacement plethysomgraph), we found out what spectacular results that one workout produced! While Tim's bodyweight actually did go down a pound, his muscle weight went up by 9.3 pounds and his body fat decreased by 9.8 pounds, resulting in a dramatic and very positive change in his physical appearance. In addition, this peak in muscle gain occurred on Day 6 of the study—i.e., six days after his workout and during which time he did *nothing* at all, which is exactly what was required for his body to produce the new muscle growth—after first being stimulated into producing more growth by the Max Contraction workout.

While I will outline the exact workout that Tim employed to stimulate such dramatic gains in muscle mass shortly, it will benefit the reader to first learn something about the protocol that Tim employed, so that the workout, when it is finally presented, will be done within a more meaningful context.

The "Max Contraction System" is a system of training that is based upon the premise that muscles perform work by shortening (i.e., contracting), and are engaged maximally when maximally contracted. Moreover, muscles are very much stronger in their position of full contraction than they are when they are extended (i.e., not fully contracted), with the result that they are capable of contracting against much heavier weights. As heavier weights require more energy to contract against than do lighter weights, the energy reserves in the muscles are taxed maximally by a maximum contraction against a maximum load. And as conventional so-called "full-range" contractions, wherein a muscle is made to go from a full stretch to a full contraction, require the trainee to lift a muscle through its weakest range of motion to get into the fully contracted or maximum contraction position, the load is substantially lighter than the muscle is able to contract against if it were simply made to perform the contraction in its strongest or maximum contraction position. The lighter load serves to minimize the stimulus and the energy drain on the muscles—the opposite of what we are trying to accomplish. The heavier the weight a muscle can be made to contract against, the more muscle fibers will be recruited to produce the force necessary to contract against it. Remember: the strongest position in a muscle's range of movement is the position of full or maximum contraction.

This fully contracted position is then maintained. Why? Because to move out of it would require moving the muscle into a position other than *maximum* and the load would have to be lightened considerably, which, again, would diminish muscle fiber and energy involvement. And while there is no motion, technically speaking, during this type of exercise, there are two measurable factors—load and time. Physiology has revealed that when a muscle is made to contract so intensely that it can only sustain such activity for one to sixty seconds (within what

The heavier the weight a muscle can be made to contract against, the more muscle fibers will be recruited to produce the force necessary to contract against it.

are called the anaerobic pathways), the stimulus for strength and size is much greater than if you train a muscle longer than this prescribed time period. To train a muscle longer than this requires training at a lower energy output so that you can pace yourself to last longer—which means lighter weights and less energy drain. Again, the opposite of what we're trying to achieve. The idea is "Max," or maximum, stimulation, not minimum stimulation.

To stimulate maximum increases in strength and muscle mass on a "per workout basis" you'll have to take each and every set you do for a given body part to the point where 100 percent of your momentary ability has been utilized. Intensity, as Mike Mentzer properly defined it, is the percentage of possible momentary muscular effort that one is capable

The position of full (or Max) contraction is the one position in a muscle's range of motion where all of its fibers can be fully activated.

of generating—with low intensity activities such as walking, light weight training, and the game of golf itself representing the lower end of the spectrum, and Max Contraction representing the other end of the spectrum. At the low end of this spectrum is the minimal percentage of possible momentary effort, while at the high end is the maximal percentage of possible momentary effort. Endeavoring to make the intensity of your exercises higher and higher is, quite simply, the most important factor influencing the rate at which you will gain strength and size.

Training to what has been labeled "the point of failure," where another second of a maximal contraction cannot be sustained despite your greatest effort will ensure that you've passed the "threshold of intensity"; i.e., the point in a set below which growth is not stimulated and above which it is. It is essential when embarking on a system such as Max Contraction to understand the basic physiological principles of exercise that are elucidated in my book *Max Contraction Training: The Scientifically Proven Method for Building Muscle Mass in Minimum Time*, particularly principles such as the "all or none" principle of muscle fiber contraction.

In reading from page 53 of the textbook *The Physiology of Exercise*, by Herbert A. DeVries of the University of Southern California, we see that:

> If muscle fiber (or motor unit) is stimulated by a single impulse at or above threshold value, it responds by a contraction, or twitch, that is maximal for any given set of conditions of nutrition, temperature, etc. In other words, stimulation by impulses much larger than threshold value will result in no increase in either the shortening or the force of contraction. The muscle fiber contracts maximally, or it does not contract at all, and this fact is referred to as the *all-or-none law* of muscle contraction.

Professor DeVries goes on to mention that "this law applies to the motor unit [a group of muscle fibers], since all its component fibers are innervated by the same nerve fiber and impulse—it does not, of course, apply to whole muscles." This principle or physiologic "law" refers to the fact that when a given muscle fiber is stimulated to contract, it will contract maximally while the rest of its fibers do not contract at all—

this as opposed to an entire muscle's fibers contracting all at once but to a lesser degree. With this in mind, it stands to reason that the surest way to involve more muscle fibers in a given contraction is to take the muscle you're training into the one position where the maximum number of muscle fibers are capable of being activated, and a sufficient load or resistance is applied to ensure that they are, in fact, called into play.

In a conventional set in which a weight is lifted up and down, one starts a given movement against, literally, "zero" contraction, then moves into a position of mild contraction, then moves into a position of greater contraction and, finally, moves into a position of maximum contraction, it is only this final position—the fully contracted position—that yields the most benefit in terms of involving the most fibers. And ironically, this position is seldom—if ever—emphasized in conventional training methods.

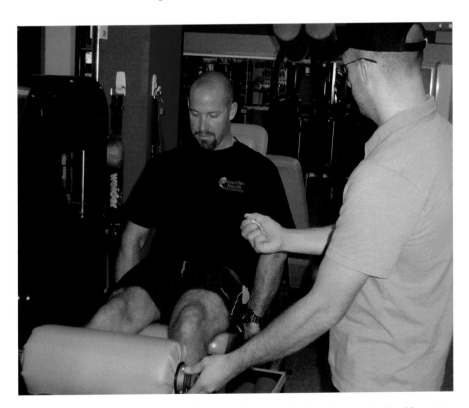

The fully contracted position of the leg extension exercise is seldom emphasized in most conventional training protocols, and yet it is the one position where the optimal amount of growth stimulation takes place.

A perfect example of this is in the leg extension exercise. Looked at physiologically, this exercise will see the trainee initiate the movement using only the barest amount of muscle fibers required to do the job. At the halfway point, a few more muscle fibers will have been called into play and then, at the position of full muscular contraction or where the legs are fully extended, as many fibers as can possibly be recruited will be activated to hold the resistance in this fully contracted position. However, long before the fibers have been stressed maximally, the resistance is typically lowered (often dropped), giving the momentarily stressed quadriceps muscles a chance to disengage (and recover to a certain extent), which is the very opposite of what you should be trying to accomplish.

This means, in effect, that in a given ten rep set performed at a typical cadence of taking two seconds to raise, one second to hold, and three seconds to lower—which lasts about sixty seconds—maximum muscular contraction takes place for a total of only six seconds. So out of a possible sixty seconds worth of maximum muscle contraction, the trainee is obtaining only one tenth of the results he is capable of deriving from the movement. Viewed in this light, it becomes painfully obvious that the trainee is wasting the other nine-tenths of the time he's been employing on the exercise. Conversely, when a given muscle group is brought into the fully contracted position and made to contract maximally against a heavy resistance for anywhere between one and sixty seconds, the maximum amount of muscle fibers and muscular energy (i.e., glycogen) that can be activated to assist in the task will be called into play until they are incapable of sustaining the maximum contraction. As soon as the trainee can no longer sustain the contraction, he will have effectively exhausted all of the muscle fibers and the energy substrates that fuel them involved in that contraction, which just so happens to be all of them.

And the sixty-second time frame is purely for purposes of illustrating the difference in efficiency between conventional or full-range training protocols and Max Contraction—or 10 percent efficiency versus 100 percent efficiency. In truth, research has indicated that only one to six seconds of maximal intensity stimulation is necessary—if the muscle is in the fully contracted position; training closer to one minute requires activating the body's aerobic system to some degree, thus compromising the pure anaerobic element—which is the element most responsible for size and strength gains.

When I first tested the system in the late 1980s, the standard time frame I implemented was forty-five to sixty seconds, which is the same time frame that Tim Peake employed—and very good gains were reported. I personally supervised the training of two subjects in 2001 who trained one day a week on a Max Contraction program of one forty-five to sixty second set of five different exercises. This averaged out to a total time frame of between 3 minutes and 45 seconds and 5 minutes total of training time per week. At the end of five weeks, the subjects had improved a minimum of 80 percent over their starting levels of strength in all exercises and, more importantly for our purposes, their lean body mass increase was a total of sixteen pounds each—and these were not untrained subjects. When you try to remember the last time that you gained sixteen pounds of pure muscle tissue over a five-week period, you'll begin to appreciate just how effective the Max Contraction System is!

Nevertheless, there was room for refinement; in the early 1990s, I experimented with increasing the resistance, which necessitated a decrease in the time of contraction (or TOC) to fifteen to thirty seconds per set—and the strength of all trainees using the revised protocol increased markedly. Finally, in 2001, after reviewing a series of physiology studies conducted over fifty years ago—particularly the studies of Muller and Hettinger, which indicated that a one-to-six second maximal contraction could produce strength gains equal to or better than protocols involving more sets and longer hold times—I decided to revise the protocol again once more increasing the intensity of the contraction by increasing the resistance and reducing the time of contraction to a mere one to six seconds. Doing so meant that the actual volume or length of the workout was reduced commensurately to only five to thirty seconds of actual workout time. Once again, the strength and size gains of those who tried the new protocol increased—and dramatically! One subject increased his shrug weight by over 400 pounds in a little less than one month of workouts performed once weekly and lasting, on average, thirty seconds each.

However, I have found that the thirty- to sixty-second time frame is a good starting point for people with Max Contraction Training as it better trains the neuromuscular pathways of the trainee, thus making him or her more efficient at recruiting muscle fibers and acclimating the trainee to the phenomenon of what genuine contractile "failure" is. It is too easy to quit during a set because of the pain associated with lactic acid build up. It is also not uncommon for a trainee to start out too heavy with too short a TOC (Time of Contraction), which results in the trainee quitting prematurely before optimal fiber recruitment and stimulation has taken place, thereby compromising his results. By gradually reducing the TOC over a period of time, the trainee is more accustomed to the protocol, his neuromuscular efficiency is enhanced, and he is more likely to terminate a set owing to legitimately being

In Max Contraction Training you don't count "repetitions," you count the number of seconds that the targeted muscle group is placed under the load.

unable to sustain a maximal muscular contraction. My recommendation would be to spend the first five months at thirty to sixty seconds of TOC, the next three to four months at a fifteen- to thirty-second TOC, and, finally, thereafter attempting to reach muscular failure with a TOC of between one and six seconds.

The reason why virtually all subjects who have used this protocol experience such dramatic improvement in strength and muscular mass is this: any exercise performed the conventional way (i.e., utilizing repetitions) involves movement either into or out of a position of maximum contraction. As maximum muscular contraction is our objective, anything less than a maximum contraction is less efficient in stimulating muscle fibers into growth. Whether the movement is performed either eccentrically or concentrically, the very fact that it moves at all means that it will have fluctuating levels of fiber involvement and, hence, fiber stimulation. Remember, the closer a movement is to the fully contracted position (that is, a movement in which maximal resistance is truly in a position of full muscular contraction), the more muscle fibers are involved and activated by the stressor. And, as we've seen, in Max, or fully contracted, exercise, all available muscle fibers are under a constant stress or "intensity" of the highest order from the moment the contraction is initiated until its completion.

In order to derive the most benefit from Max Contraction Training, it is vitally important to select exercises that allow you to achieve a full muscular contraction. Many conventional and popular bodybuilding exercises do not incorporate the proper physics to provide maximum resistance in the fully contracted position. I'm thinking here of movements such as squats, barbell curls (where the resistance falls off once you pass through the halfway point of the movement), and most types of pressing movements.

It is this lack of direct resistance in the fully contracted position that makes these exercises inefficient in a Max Contraction Training program. Exercises must be selected for Max Contraction Training that enable the targeted muscle group to be contracted maximally against a maximum resistance for a thirty- to sixty-second time period. The following is a list of exercises that we put Tim Peake on during the Nautilus North study and have been found to be the best for this purpose.

What follows is the exact program that Tim used (exercises, weights, and contraction times):

Tim Peake Workout

Exercise	Weight (in pounds)	Time of Contraction (in seconds)
Hip and Back	170	49
Leg Extension	220	40
Leg Curl	90	36
Multi-Exercise (Calf Raise)	180	42
Super Pullover (Lats)	190	45
Lower Back	260	37
Ten Degree Chest	160	37
Lateral Raise	170	45
Triceps Kickbacks	70	46
Multi Biceps	140	41
Nautilus Ab	180	35

Now it should be pointed out that Tim Peake also has good genetics, which means that it might take him longer to exhaust his muscular reserves than the average person. For anybody starting out I would recommend cutting Tim's workout in half, performing Exercises 1 through 6 in one workout, and then performing Exercises 7 through 11 after one week's rest. The two workouts should then be alternated with seven (or more) days in between.

How the exercises are performed

Hip and Back:
While lying on the back, position the body so that the hips are aligned with the axes of the cam. Extend both legs and push back with the arms until the legs, with the feet together, are locked at the knees and below parallel to

the floor so as to arch the back. Either push out or have a training partner push the resistance arms down until both legs are joined at extension. Arch the back and contract the buttocks. Sustain this contraction for 30 to 60 seconds.

Leg Extensions:
Assume a properly aligned position in the machine. Extend both legs smoothly as far as possible (you may require a training partner to help you lift the resistance into the fully contracted position). Sustain this contraction for 30 to 60 seconds.

Leg Curl:
Lie face down on the machine with the heels placed under the rollers. The knees should be just off the bench. Lightly grasp handles. Curl legs (or have your training partner assist in raising the movement arm for you) trying to touch heels

to buttocks. Lift buttocks at the top of the movement to increase the muscle contraction. Pause in this fully contracted position for 30 to 60 seconds.

Multi-Exercise (Calf Raise):
Affix the weight belt around your waist and stand up straight. Place your hands on the cross carriage in front of you and step onto the first step of the Multi-Exercise machine. Raise yourself up, using only the

strength of your calf muscles), onto your tiptoes until your calves are fully contracted. Sustain this contraction for 30 to 60 seconds.

Super Pullover:
Adjust seat so that the shoulder rotates on a common axis with the cam. Assume upright position and fasten seat belt tightly. Press foot pedal until elbow pads are about chin level (you may require a training partner's assistance) and place elbows on pads. Hands

should be open and resting on the curved portion of bar. Remove legs from pedal and slowly rotate elbows down until they are level with the lower portion of your chest. Sustain this contraction for 30 to 60 seconds.

Lower Back:
Enter the lower back machine by straddling the seat bottom. Sit forward in seat. Make sure that your back is underneath the

highest roller pad. Stabilize your lower body by moving your thighs under the roller pads. Adjust the pads until your thighs are secure. Place feet firmly on platform or step and fasten the seat belt. Interlace your fingers across your waist and move your torso backward smoothly and slowly until it is in line with thighs. Sustain this fully contracted position for 30 to 60 seconds.

Ten Degree Chest Machine:
Lie on your back with your head higher than your hips. Place your arms under the roller pads. The pads should be in the crooks of your elbows. Move both arms (with the help of a training partner if necessary) in a rotary fashion until the roller pads touch over your chest. Sustain this fully contracted position for 30 to 60 seconds.

Double Shoulder (Lateral Raise):
Adjust the seat so that the shoulder joints are in line with axes of the cam. Fasten seat belt and pull hands back until knuckles touch pads. Lead with elbows and raise both arms

(again, with the assistance of a training partner if necessary) until parallel with floor. Sustain this full contraction for between 30 and 60 seconds.

Triceps Kickbacks:
Sit down in the Super Pullover machine and adjust the seat so that the shoulder rotates on a common axis with the cam. Assume an upright position and fasten the seat belt tightly. Press foot pedal until elbow pads are about chin level (you may require a training partner's assistance) and place elbows on pads. Your hands should be hanging down at your sides and not resting on the bar. Remove legs from pedal and draw your elbows back so that your lower arms are behind the body at either side of your torso. Sustain this contraction for 30 to 60 seconds.

Biceps Curl:
In a seated position, place elbows on pad aligned with center of cams. Adjust seat so that shoulders are lower than elbows. Curl both arms until wrists are just in front of neck. Sustain this fully contracted position for between 30 and 60 seconds.

Abdominal Machine:
Assume a properly aligned position. Spread knees and sit erect. Shorten the distance between your ribcage and navel by contracting your abdominal muscles only. If necessary, have a training partner assist you into the position of full contraction of the abdominals. Do not pull with latissimus or triceps muscles. Keep legs relaxed. Sustain this fully contracted position for between 30 and 60 seconds.

Purpose and benefits of this program

Nautilus Machine	Muscles Developed	Action of Muscles	Fitness Basis for Exercise
Hip and Back	Buttocks, lower back	Extend the spine, flexion of the spine, extend upper leg	Eliminates lower back-related problems.
Leg Extension	Quadriceps	Extend lower leg	Eliminates frontal thigh pulls
Leg Curl	Hamstrings	Extend and flex upper leg, flex lower leg	Eliminates rear thigh pulls
Calf Raise	Calves	Raise the heel	Assists in protecting the joints of the ankle and knee
Pullover	Latissimus dorsi	Move arm down and backward, stabilize torso	Eliminates lat pulls, stabilizes shoulder
Lower Back	Spinal erector muscles	Draw trunk to an upright position	Prevents lower back strain, stabilizes spine
Ten Degree Chest Pull	Chest	Draw arm across torso	Eliminate chest pulls, stabilizes shoulder
Lateral Raise	Deltoids (shoulder)	Raise, lower, and rotate shoulder	Eliminates shoulder-related problems
Multi Biceps	Biceps	Flex the arm	Assists in holding arm comfortably at proper angle
Kickbacks	Triceps	Extend the arm	Assists in holding arm comfortably at proper angle
Abdominal	Rectus abdominus	Flex spine, stabilize posture	Assists in breathing by stabilizing rib cage

Non-Nautilus Max Contraction Workout

As not everyone will have access to the same machines (Nautilus, first generation) that Tim Peake and the other trainees in the Nautilus

North study utilized, I am presenting as an alternative a Max Contraction workout using conventional equipment that can also be employed with excellent results. The key is to train once every seven days and to take each set to the point where you can no longer sustain the maximum contraction.

Max Contraction workout

1. Quads: Leg extensions
2. Hams: Leg curls
3. Calves: Donkey calf raise
4. Lats and Pecs: Pulldowns (using Max Straps)
5. Traps: Shrugs
6. Delts: Lateral raises
7. Pecs: Pec deck
8. Triceps: Max Straps pushdown or dumbbell kickbacks
9. Biceps: Flexed arm hang
10. Forearms: Wrist curls
11. Abs: Crunches

The following section outlines the correct way to perform each exercise.

Leg Extensions:
Sit down on a leg extension machine and place your feet behind the roller pads so that your knees are snug against the seat. Keeping your head and shoulders straight, slowly straighten both legs until you reach the fully contracted position and hold for a full 30 to 60 seconds. Immediately move on to your next exercise.

Leg Curls:
Lie face down on the leg curl machine and place your feet

under the roller pads with your knees just over the edge of the bench and slowly curl your lower legs up until they're almost touching your buttocks. Once in this fully contracted position, hold the contraction for a full 30 to 60 seconds.

Standing Calf Raises:
Step underneath the shoulder pads of a standing calf raise machine so that the balls of your feet are on the block and your heels are almost touching the ground. From this position of full stretch, slowly contract your gastrocnemius (or calf muscles) until your calves are fully contracted. Hold this fully contracted position for 30 to 60 seconds before lowering the resistance fully and rushing on to your next exercise.

Pulldowns (using Max Straps):

This exercise emphasizes several muscle groups, most notably the latissimus dorsi, the biceps, the triceps, the rear deltoids, the trapezius, the pectorals (pec minor especially), and the abdominals. To begin this exercise, position yourself in a lat pulldown machine and insert your arms through the Max Straps so that the bottom padded part of the strap is over the end of your upper arm (nearest the elbow joint) and your hands are resting against the side straps. Don't close your hands on the straps, as this will unnecessarily involve and fatigue the forearm muscles and (to a lesser extent) the biceps. Using only the strength of your latissimus dorsi muscles, draw your elbows down and back until they are just to the sides of your lower ribs. Hold for 30 to 60 seconds. Once the weights start piling up, you will need assistance to bring your elbows down into the fully contracted position, as your holding strength is always stronger than your positive or concentric strength.

Shrugs:

Do not make the mistake of allowing your ego to dictate your poundage in this exercise. Form should always take precedence over

weight for the simple fact
that if your muscles aren't
responsible for moving the
weight, they will not be
adequately stimulated. It
will, however, be possible
to handle some fairly heavy
weight in this exercise as
your trapezius muscles
are among the strongest
in the body. To perform
this exercise, grab hold of

the handles on a Universal bench press machine, a Hammer shrug
machine, or a barbell and stand erect so that the barbell (if you are
using a barbell) is directly in front of your thighs. Slowly begin to
contract your traps so that your shoulders ascend up towards the
ceiling. When the weight has been raised as high as it can go, hold
the contraction for a full 30 to 60 seconds.

Lateral Raises:
This exercise effectively isolates and stimulates the lateral head of
the deltoid to help to stabilize your shoulder joint and to increase

strength in all movements requiring lateral flexion of the shoulder. Take hold of a pair of dumbbells. Stand up straight so that they are just in front of your thighs, with your body perfectly erect and your back straight. Smoothly with lateral head output only and with your elbows locked, begin to raise the dumbbells to a height just above shoulder level. Hold the resistance there for 30 to 60 seconds.

Max Strap Pulldowns (or Dumbell Kickbacks): With ring of the Max Straps attached to the hook at the end of an overhead pulley, push your forearms down until they are locked out and sustain this contraction for 30 to 60 seconds. If you do not have access to a set of Max Straps, you may wish to perform dumbbell kickbacks instead.

To perform this exercise, take hold of a dumbbell and bend over at the waist. Place one hand on a bench for support and, maintaining the bent-over position, draw the dumbbell behind you until your arm is as far behind your torso as you can move it and your arm is fully locked out. Sustain this maximum contraction for 30 to 60 seconds and then repeat the procedure with the opposite arm.

Flexed Arm Hang:

If you choose to perform palms-under, close-grip chins (popularly called the "flexed arm hang"), begin by standing on a chair and placing your hands on the chinning bar with an underhand palms-up grip. Assume a position where you are parallel with the top of the bar and your biceps are fully contracted. Now, easily, step off the chair until your biceps contract fully, thus holding you up. Hold—depending on your personal bodyweight and existing strength levels—for between 30 and 60 seconds.

Wrist Curls:

Take hold of a barbell with a palms-up grip and sit down at the end of a short bench. Place your wrists just over the end of your knees and slowly curl your wrists upward in a semi-circular arc toward your torso. Once you have reached this fully contracted position, sustain it for 30 to 60 seconds.

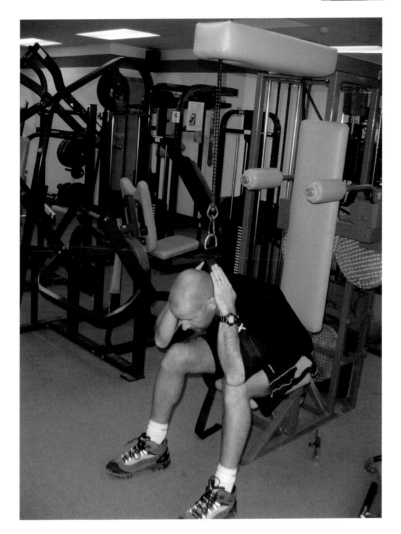

Max Strap Crunches:
Attach the Max Straps to an overhead pulley (ideally on a lat pulldown
machine that has a seat and knee pad). Sit down on the seat and place
your arms through the Max Straps so that the pads are over the bends
in your elbows. Lower your elbows down to a point and out to the
sides so that the base of the Max Straps is touching the back of your
neck. Now slowly bend your torso over while drawing your elbows
downwards until your elbows are almost touching your knees. Once
you've hit the fully contracted position, sustain it for 30 to 60 seconds.

7
TIPS FOR MORE PRODUCTIVE WORKOUTS

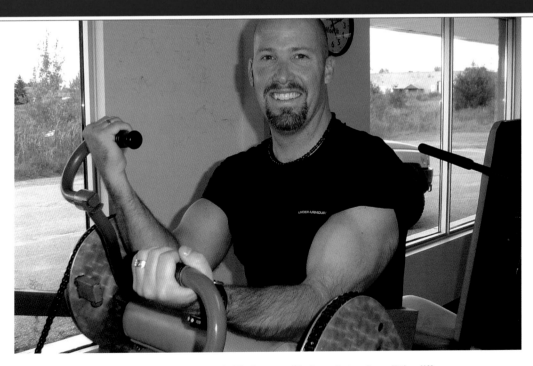

Simply lifting weights isn't enough; it's *how* you lift them that makes all the difference.

I n supervising the workouts of thousands of trainees over the years, I've been able to observe what things trainees can do to help maximize their results. Sometimes it's the little things that can make the difference, particularly when employing a powerful protocol such as Max Contraction. Here is a list of tips that will ensure that your workouts are as productive as possible:

Longer time of contraction (TOC) for beginners

If you are a beginner to strength training or, indeed, if you are an experienced trainee who is a beginner to Max Contraction Training, you will be well served if, during your first four to six months of working out, you hold each contraction for thirty to sixty seconds. This

Beginners should employ a Time of Contraction (TOC) in the 30-60-second range.

longer hold time will serve to develop greater neuromuscular efficiency and help to better acclimate you to the new training protocol. After your first four to six months of working out, however, you should increase the intensity by increasing the resistance and reducing your TOC to six seconds or less.

Keep accurate records

Learning and advancement are almost always reached through trial and error. By making a trial and missing the mark and then noting the error, you can make proper adjustments and move on toward the goal. A training logbook will

Precise record keeping is a must. It allows you to measure (and thus determine) if your previous workout had the desired effect of making you stronger.

prove invaluable in this regard. Keeping a record of every proper turn (as well as every mistake—such as training too frequently) can help you avoid the pitfalls that will slow you down. A logbook serves as a record of workouts and should include daily calorie intake (including the types of foods), the weights used in each exercises, the TOC for each exercise, and the total weight lifted (TWL), which is the total weight, taken as an aggregate, of all the exercises you performed in a given workout. These figures (in particular the TWL), will allow you to know at a glance whether you are progressing in your efforts, plateauing, or even regressing—sure indicators of progress, inadequate recovery, and overtraining, respectively. By also recording your daily food consumption, you can calculate your nutritional requirements for future weight gain and loss as well as observe the effects of certain diets on moods, training drive, and progress. Experimenting with different weights, contraction times, and charting your progress can yield invaluable training data. Eventually you'll have enough information in your journal to make precise determinations.

Proceed cautiously

If you do not have a training partner you must exercise caution when commencing any exercise using Max Contraction; i.e., lift the resistance slowly (so as not to damage any ligaments or muscle tissue) into the position of full-muscular contraction, just as you would if you were performing a regular set. However, instead of lowering the resistance, you will hold this fully contracted position for a minimum of thirty seconds and a maximum of sixty. If you can hold the resistance longer than sixty seconds, it's too light to be maximally effective and you should heavy it up by 5 percent or so for your next workout. If you can't hold the resistance for thirty seconds, then it's too heavy and you should reduce the resistance by 5 percent until you can contract the muscle against the resistance for one full second.

Training partners

If you do train with a partner (or two) who can lift the weight into the fully contracted position for you, make sure he or she (or they) don't simply "drop" the weight into your control once you're in the fully contracted position as the sudden shock to the joint of articulation could prove traumatic. Every movement must be performed slowly, particularly the settling into the fully contracted position.

Understand the nature of high energy exercise

You may notice that as your muscles fatigue they will begin to shake (sometimes rather violently) at the thirty to sixty

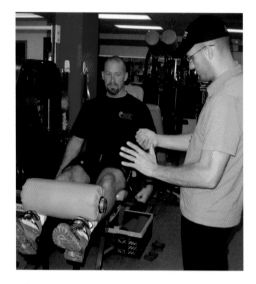

A good personal trainer who understands the physiology of the process will prove invaluable to the success of your workouts.

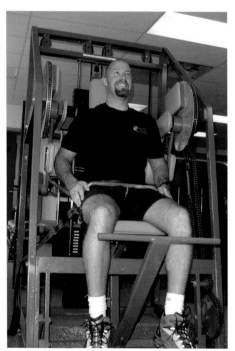

Training through a full range of motion is neither necessary nor desirable.

second mark—but this is as it should be. It's simply an indicator that your muscles are firing more and more fibers to maintain the contraction and burning up more energy. Remember, the more energy they use, the greater the growth stimulation will be. After a Max Contraction workout, you will feel like your limbs are made of jelly owing to the high volume of energy you will have expended. At which point you will be entering the stage of recovery and growth, requiring you to rest completely (i.e., take part in no other form of strenuous exercise) until your next workout a minimum of seven days later.

Allow sufficient time for adequate recovery and growth to take place

Beginners to Max Contraction Training should structure their workouts seven days apart. Intermediates should structure their workouts such that they are training but once every eight to ten days, while advanced trainees should train no more than once every fourteen days.

Always try to increase the resistance your muscles are made to contract against, try to extend the time that you are able to contract against a given load—or both—each and every workout.

Strive to increase the intensity

Always strive for increased intensity via additional seconds of contraction until a full sixty seconds has been obtained, at which point you can increase the resistance imposed on the muscle group and aim for thirty seconds again. If you continue to do this, you will be rewarded for your efforts with the best gains of your golfing career.

8
ADVANCED TRAINING

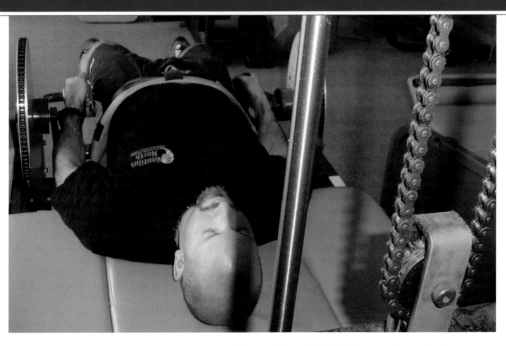

As a trainee grows stronger, the stresses he can bring to his body increase dramatically—
and must be compensated for.

A s an individual grows stronger, the energy demands he places upon his body grow greater. Consider the following two workouts:

Exercise	Workout 1	Workout 2
Leg Extension	80 pounds/30 seconds	150 pounds/55 seconds
Leg Curl	50 pounds/30 seconds	90 pounds/60 seconds
Standing Calf Raise	130 pounds/30 seconds	250 pounds/50 seconds
Max Straps Pulldown	120 pounds/30 seconds	220 pounds/60 seconds
Pec Deck	50 pounds/35 seconds	130 pounds/60 seconds
Machine Lateral Raise	25 pounds/30 seconds	70 pounds/60 seconds
Flexed Arm Hang	Bodyweight (150)/ 25 seconds	Bodyweight (159) + 30 pounds/ 45 seconds
Max Straps Kickback	50 pounds/37 seconds	120 pounds/60 seconds
Crunches	60 pounds/30 seconds	110 pounds/60 seconds

These are workout charts from the same client over a three-month period. The exercises, and the sequence in which they were performed, are identical. What has changed is the amount of weight he was able to have his muscles contract against and the time that he was able to sustain those contractions. Workout 1 saw him lift a total of 715 pounds for a total of 4 minutes and 37 seconds. Workout 2 saw him lift a total of 1,299 pounds for a total of 8 minutes and 30 seconds. The energy required to lift 1,299 pounds worth of weight is obviously greater than the energy required to lift 715 pounds (by 584 pounds) and to contract against this resistance for 4 minutes and 7 seconds longer, likewise requires a greater energy output from his muscles. Consequently, the amount of time required to put back into the body the energy that he expended in getting his muscles to contract against 1,299 pounds for 8 minutes and 30 seconds will be longer than it would with any lesser amount of weight and time. In other words, your "battery" doesn't get bigger, but the drain on it from your stronger muscles gets greater and greater with every trip to the gym (or at least it should if your training is producing strength gains).

This last point is vital to grasp for the trainee who has already attained a certain level of development and strength and wishes to progress further, closer to the limits of his or her genetic potential.

What the individual will find is that he is able to drain his muscles so much more thoroughly now that he simply runs out of gas after two or three exercises. Using our illustration above, if it initially required nine exercises, 715 pounds and 4 minutes and 37 seconds of effort to drain the muscles of 100 percent of their energy, within three months of exercising once a week, this same individual is now capable of moving that same amount of weight and draining that same 100 percent of energy with only four exercises and roughly 3 minutes and 40 seconds worth of exercise.

There are two types of energy utilized by the body when producing physiological change. One is the glycogen that is stored on-site with each muscle group (and that replenishes rather quickly), and the other has been referred to as "adaptation energy," a more non-specific systemic energy, that takes a considerably longer time to replenish.

The late Dr. Hans Selye, one of the world's pioneers in stress research, was the first to label this deeper energy source "adaptation energy," and it is this energy that must be tapped or called upon for the advanced trainee to continue to make gains in strength and lean tissue mass. According to Selye, this adaptation energy is something quite apart from caloric energy, being inherited by each individual upon his birth, and its existence—and hence our adaptive (or muscle growth) capacity—is not infinite:

> Although we have no precise scientific method for measuring adaptation energy, experiments with laboratory animals offer rather convincing evidence that the capacity for adaptation is finite. Our reserves of adaptation energy could be compared to an inherited fortune from which we can make withdrawals; but there is no proof that we can also make additional deposits. We can

squander our adaptability recklessly, "burning the candle at both ends," or we can learn to make this valuable resource last long, by using it wisely and sparingly, only for things that are worthwhile and cause least distress.

As I have said, we have no objective proof that additional deposits of adaptation energy can be made beyond that inherited from our parents. Yet, everyone knows from personal experience that, after complete exhaustion by excessively stressful work during the day, a good night's sleep—and, after even more severe exhaustion, a few weeks of restful holidays—can restore our resistance and adaptability very close to what it was before. . . . If this is the case, we must distinguish between *superficial* and *deep* adaptation energy. Superficial adaptation energy is immediately available upon demand, like money in a bank account that is readily accessible by writing out a check. On the other hand, deep adaptation energy is stored away safely as a reserve, just as part of our inherited fortune may be invested in stocks and bonds, which must first be sold to replenish our checking account, thus furnishing another supply of immediately usable cash. Still, after a lifetime of constant expenditure, even our last investments will be eventually exhausted if we only spend and never earn.

And this is why as you grow stronger, and your ability to exhaust this energy grows greater, you must reduce the volume and frequency of your workouts. If you attempt to train for longer periods of time—"burning the candle at both ends," as Selye points out—then only the superficial adaptation energy is employed, but, over time, this will lead to a gradual draining of your deep reserves of adaptation energy, which could otherwise go to cover your energy debt of superficial adaptation energy. This is energy "squandered recklessly," as all of your adaptation energy will have been used up—not in the creation of stronger and bigger muscles, but in cultivating an ability to tolerate longer workouts. Use this energy "wisely" (specifically for the adaptation of size and strength) and "sparingly" (with short bursts of intense training performed infrequently). Prudent use will assure that it goes exclusively toward building larger and stronger muscles.

And as you grow stronger, the reality is that you simply run out of gas sooner in your workouts, which means that your workouts must be abbreviated in a manner that will continue to provide adequate stimulation to all the major muscle groups of the body while your body still has sufficient energy to invest in the exercises. How abbreviated? We recently completed another study at Nautilus North that was conducted with the primary objective of having clients lose body fat and establishing the role of building muscle in raising subjects' basal metabolic rate, thus burning calories at a greater rate, twenty-four hours a day, seven days a week.

The subjects for this study were twenty-two women and eleven men (aged twenty-five to sixty-four). The study lasted ten weeks. No supplements or special dietary restrictions were imposed, save for using a well-balanced but modestly reduced calorie diet in conjunction with a workout that lasted a mere two minutes and was performed but once a week. Here are the results:

Weight and Fat Losses

Total Weight Loss:	442.4 lbs
Greatest Weight Loss (Men):	43.2 lbs
Greatest Weight Loss (Women):	25.8 lbs
Average Weight Loss:	17.02 lbs
Total Pure Fat Loss:	405 lbs
Greatest Fat Loss (Men):	33.8 lbs
Average Fat Loss (Men):	20.9 lbs
Greatest Fat Loss (Women):	23.6 lbs
Average Fat Loss (Women):	13.2 lbs
Average Pure Fat Loss:	15.58 lbs

Strength Increase (After Ten Workouts)

Lower Body (Men):	43.05%
Upper Body (Men):	30.42%
Lower Body (Women):	43.73%
Upper Body (Women):	32.51%
Average Overall Strength Increase:	35.46%
Average Lean Gain % (Men):	+6.21%

Average Lean Gain % (Women):   +4.52%
Total Lean Muscle Increase: +132.8%
Overall Average Lean Muscle Gain: +5.11%

Given that all of the subjects on this study had been training hard for over one year, this level of lean (and strength) gain is considerable. Moreover, to my knowledge, never before in the history of fat loss and exercise (and that's quite a history) has there ever been this much fat loss from this little amount of exercise—and all of the above results were achieved employing a workout that lasted (on average) a mere two minutes and was performed *only once a week*! Moreover, when the results were compared between groups that trained with more exercise versus those that trained with less, that those who trained the least lost more fat and gained more muscle by a ratio of two to one! No forty-five-minute per day sessions on a treadmill were necessary—nor any other form of aerobic exercise.

Knowing this, think for a moment of the billions of man-hours that have been wasted over the years by people who believe they "have to" train several hours a week if they wish to lose body fat.

In terms of diet, the subjects on the study consumed regular food—three meals a day, plus two snacks; food that you can find in any supermarket. No drugs were involved. No supplements were employed, nor were they required. And, in case you were wondering, we are halfway through another round of this program, this time with sixty-five subjects—and ALL of them are repeating the results of those on the first study.

Health benefits

That's all well and good for body fat loss—but what about health benefits? This is where even we were quite surprised at the results. Given the high incidence of injury and the occurrence of osteoarthritis from over-use of joints and connective tissues, it is questionable that the present trend of performing "more" exercise outweighs its health risks. The ideal health prescription would be to perform the precise amount of exercise required, rather than trying to determine just how much exercise you can tolerate. The health benefits of our fat loss program were nothing short of remarkable. Blood pressure medications were found to be no longer necessary (a sure sign of cardiovascular improvement) for 30 percent of the subjects who took part in the study; cholesterol medications were also found to be no longer necessary for the same 30 percent, and individuals who had been diagnosed with diabetes were found to require 70 percent less insulin—that's right, not a little less, but 70 percent less! Individuals who had come off of knee replacement surgery now found that they could literally bound up flights of stairs that otherwise had represented an insurmountable obstacle. Incredible results from a workout that lasted a fraction of the time that most individuals seeking to lose weight follow.

The reason?

In a word: science. In the past, individuals seeking to lose weight have looked to the suspect opinion of the fitness industry which exists to sell services and products, not to dispense valid scientific information (particularly when it is this simple). Consider the following medical facts:

- Muscle is metabolically expensive tissue. It requires more calories at rest than any other tissue and is responsible for 70 percent of the calories burned on a daily basis. The more you have of it, the higher your resting metabolic rate (fat burning ability) will be.
- Muscle is the first casualty on most diets and on most exercise programs. If you do not use resistance exercise, you will lose muscle. If you use resistance exercise, but it is performed for too many exercises or too often, you will—again—lose muscle tissue.
- To build muscle, it must be trained within its anaerobic pathways (up to 70 seconds). Any training beyond this point dilutes the potency of the training stimulus and could cost you muscle.
- Training too frequently prevents your body from producing or even maintaining muscle tissue.

While the above facts have been known by exercise scientists for over fifty years, they have never been applied to people's fat loss aspirations—until this program. The dramatic success of this program has resulted in it being added as a permanent part of the Nautilus North program.

A one-set workout?

During the ten-week Nautilus North/Body Comp fat loss program we recognized that the clients would have to train as intensely as they could in order to preserve (and hopefully) increase their lean tissue levels during a negative calorie balance. Doing so would lead to an increased metabolic rate and cause them to burn more calories—even while at rest—at a more rapid rate. As it is true that the greater the intensity of effort, the briefer such effort can be, we quickly recognized that some clients were "out of gas" after performing only two sets in their weekly workouts. As a result, during the course of the study we created two groups. One group was kept at three exercises (performed once a week), while the training volume of the other group was reduced to a mere two sets (performed once a week). The results? The group that did less training (the two sets once a week group), gained more muscle and lost more fat—by a two to one ratio! This wasn't an anomaly either, but rather the normal response for everyone right across the board. One of the clients in the two sets once a week group indicated that she was willing to experiment in reducing the volume of her workout even further. After the study had completed, she agreed to drop her weekly workout down from two sets to one high-intensity set per session performed but once a week. After four more weeks on a reduced calorie diet, and training on average for one minute per week, we re-tested her in the Bod Pod body composition tracking machine. We were stunned to learn that such a brief workout had resulted in her losing an additional five pounds of fat, and gaining an additional three pounds of muscle! We have since trained another dozen people in this manner, and ALL of them are outperforming (in terms of strength gains) those who are performing more sets. We will be conducting another in-depth study of this phenomenon in the near future where all of the subjects will perform one set per week and will report the findings through the Max Contraction website (www.maxcontraction.com) at that time. Certainly the implications from this would completely revolutionize the fitness industry.

We have found that in order to make judicious use of his limited energy reserves, the advanced trainee should limit himself to three exercises:

Max Strap Pulldowns

Leg Extensions

Leg Curls

These three exercises will work all of the major muscle groups in the body, and, if they feel too taxing, then reduce the workout to two exercises, either leg extensions and leg curls together in one workout and Max Strap pulldowns in the other, or Max Strap pulldowns and leg extensions in one workout, and Max Strap pulldowns and leg curls in the other.

This will keep the volume of the workouts down to a level that will allow you give 100 percent to each exercise while you still have 100 percent to give, thus ensuring that you are doing everything within your power to continue to stimulate an adaptive response to get stronger and leaner, while keeping the workouts brief and infrequent enough (they should be performed with a minimum of seven days in between, and, as you grow stronger, push that interval out to fourteen days) to allow for the adaptive response the training stimulated to be produced.

PART THREE:

ADDITIONAL

9
WHAT ABOUT STRETCHING?

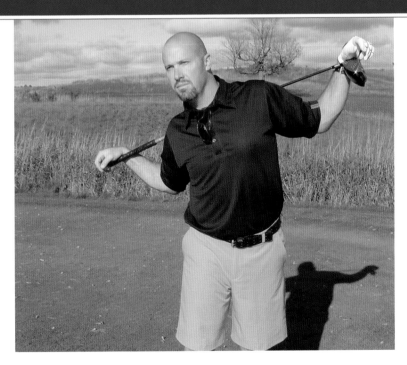

Stretching, contrary to popular belief, does not warm up the muscles prior to golfing.

Most golfers believe that stretching is a healthy thing to do. For instance, if you go to any golf course before a game or go to a driving range, you will usually see a cadre of golfers twisting their torsos with their clubs across their shoulders, or reaching down to touch their toes or performing some sort of trunk rotation to "limber up."

Most golfers believe that stretching does one or all of the following things:

1. It warms up the muscles.
2. It helps to prevent injuries.
3. It makes you more flexible.
4. It helps you to recover more quickly from an injury.
5. It makes you stronger.

All of the above five points are wrong—stretching does *none* of these things. I don't say that this is simply my opinion on the subject of stretching, but rather the conclusion of scientists and exercise physiologists who have studied stretching and its effects on the body.

Scientific research shows that stretching—the kind of stretching that the average golfer does during his workouts at the gym, or even the kind of stretching that he does on the course prior to a game—could very well be costing him several strokes and increasing his risk of injury. Articles published in recent years, reviewing hundreds of studies, have concluded that there isn't any compelling evidence that stretching prevents injury or reduces muscle soreness. Also, a study conducted in the year 2000 which looked at many hundreds of soldiers who stretched revealed no sign of benefit and even some risks to stretching.

Let's look more closely at what science has to say about each of these five common misconceptions about the alleged value of stretching:

Stretching Does Not Warm Up Muscles

You simply cannot warm up your muscles by stretching them. According to researcher Paul Ingraham, the idea that stretching will warm you up is comparable to "trying to cook a steak by pulling on it." According to Ingraham, "body heat is generated by *metabolic activity*, particularly muscle contractions. The best way to warm up is to start doing a kinder, gentler version of the activity you have in mind: walk before you run. You simply cannot warm up your muscles by stretching them."

Since stretching does not "contract" muscles, there is no metabolic activity that takes place. Stretching before your muscles are warmed up can actually increase your chance of injury. Taking a "cold" muscle and putting it in its weakest position (fully stretched) and then applying a load of sorts (either the weight of the body or, in the case of a hurdler's stretch, muscular force) is how muscles get injured.

Stretching Does Not Prevent Injuries

A study in the *British Medical Journal* in 2002 studied the effects of stretching on preventing injuries. The scientists who conducted the study concluded that "stretching before exercising does not reduce the risk of injury."

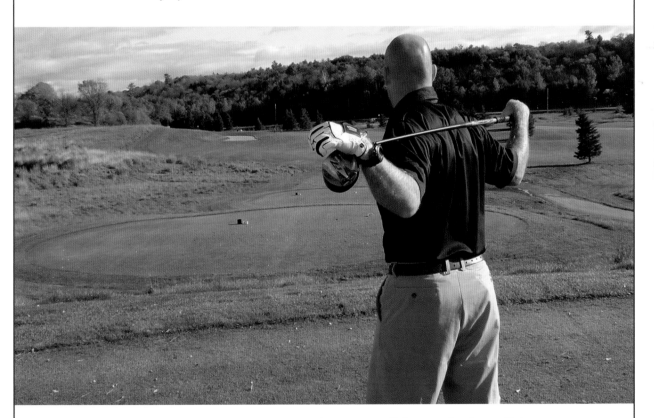

A study conducted in 2000 revealed that stretching can actually increase the chance of injury.

Research conducted at the University of Hawaii showed that stretching could actually be associated with a higher risk of injury. The study focused on runners who stretched regularly and found that they were 33 percent more likely to be injured compared to those who never stretched. In addition, a review of research by scientists in Australia also suggests that the benefits of stretching are minimal. The Australian researchers looked at five studies, three of which examined the effects of stretching performed after exercise, and two looking at stretching before exercise. These studies showed that stretching did not help to prevent injuries and it did not help to reduce soreness. Also, data taken from two studies of army recruits in training, whose risk of injury is high, showed that muscle stretching would serve to prevent an injury, on average, on one person—every twenty-three years. As most athletes are exposed to lower risks of injury—compared to soldiers—the remote benefit of stretching is believed to be even lower than this.

Stretching Does Not Make You More Flexible

Muscles have a limited range over which they can be stretched—in order for the muscles, and the joints they serve, to be protected. Most people have a normal range of motion—which is why it's called "normal." You can only stretch as far as your muscles will allow you—and attempting to stretch beyond your limitations can be dangerous, as it results in a weakening of the tendons and ligaments. Unless you are specifically frustrated because you lack sufficient range of motion in a joint to perform a task, you probably don't need to be more flexible. Fred Hahn, a top personal trainer and fitness authority from New York mentions in his online article "What is Flexibility?" that:

> Our ability to voluntarily move our joints is entirely dependent upon muscular strength. (Without muscles we couldn't move at all.) This being the case, what good does it do us to have marionette-like joints if this condition is nothing more than joint instability? People who you see at parties grasping their hands behind their back or putting their head between their knees or bending over backwards like a pretzel are demonstrating an unusual degree of joint laxity that is largely genetically inherited. (Harry Houdini,

the great escape artist, is a perfect example of this.) Though we may clap and marvel at their carnival-like contortions, this kind of pliability is not to be envied. On the contrary, it is to be avoided. It is not, by any stretch of the imagination (pun intended), an indication of being flexible in a positive sense. It is a warning of gross and ultimately dangerous tendon and ligament laxity.

You will not make a rubber band more elastic by continuously stretching it to its limits. At best, you eventually cause it to become permanently over stretched. The same is true for your muscles, tendons, and ligaments.

Stretching Does Not Help You Recover from an Injury More Quickly

Since stretching does not involve contraction, it does little to draw blood into a muscle. Blood is the best natural healer that the body has; it brings nutrients that assist in repairing injured tissue and removes the waste products that result from repair. Therefore, stretching does not help you to recover from an injury more quickly than not stretching. Research performed by scientists Rob D. Herbert and Michael Gabriel in Australia reveals that "stretching before or after exercising does not confer protection from muscle soreness."

Stretching Does Not Make You Stronger

Recently, a new study presented at the 2006 meeting of the American College of Sports Medicine looked into what effect stretching had on strength. Strength is important in that it allows athletes to perform with greater speed and power, and also protects the athlete from injury. The study featured eighteen college students who performed a one-rep-maximum test of knee flexion after doing zero, one, two, three, four, five or six thirty-second hamstring stretches. Just one thirty-second stretch reduced one-rep maximums by 5.4 percent. After the subjects did six thirty-second stretches, their strength declined by 12.4 percent.

So stretching—even for as little as thirty seconds—makes you weaker, not stronger. And since a golfer wants to be stronger and less susceptible to injury, stretching is not something that any rational golfer should engage in. So, if stretching is not desirable, what is a golfer to do to optimize his flexibility? The answer might surprise you—Max Contraction Training. This point is probably the most difficult to believe as flexibility has always been associated with stretching a given muscle and its joints to achieve a full, or "normal" physiological range of motion. However, it's very important to understand what flexibility really is governed by, and what factors influence its expression.

The entire body is regulated by the brain via the nervous system, and the brain is able to accomplish this tremendously complex task

Power—the kind necessary to blast out of wet sand—is not produced as a result of passive stretching.

via an elaborate feedback system that provides information about both the environment within and outside the body. This feedback system processes information, and the brain then sends directives derived from this information to all given body parts in order to properly control all the mechanisms involved with being alive. One of the most basic characteristics of life is locomotion or movement. The importance of movement expands beyond the need to get from point A to point B; movement is essential for our species' circulatory, lymphatic, and neurological functioning. Generally speaking, in terms of our musculoskeletal system, the primary function of ligaments is to connect bone to bone, which, by definition, creates a joint. This ligament tissue expands around the joint to form a joint capsule, which provides integrity and support to the joint. Muscles function primarily to move the bones to which they are attached via movement around these joints. This is what allows our bodies to move. Muscles serve a secondary function as well, which is to support and protect the joints.

Our brain receives information about the joints and muscles via tiny nerve receptors classified as mechanoreceptors. These are situated in the joint's capsules and ligaments. It is these nerve endings that give us our kinesiological awareness (the ability to know where our body parts are as they move through space without actually having to see them). For example, close your eyes and move your hands so that they move upward in front of your face and then above your head. Now, if your nervous system is functioning properly you will know without actually seeing your hand that it is either above or below your head. It is through similar receptors that other information about a given joint is relayed to the brain. If the brain is sent information from a properly functioning joint that all is well, then the brain will send out messages to the muscles that both move and support that joint that they can remain at a relatively loose resting tonus, and that it is okay to move that joint throughout its normal range of motion. If, however, there is excessive stress being placed on a joint via some mechanism (such as heavy full-range training or even occupational stress), then the message to the brain is that "all is not well," and the brain will now increase resting muscle tonus and decrease the normal range of motion as it perceived movement of that joint as further irritation.

And this biological process is, in fact, is one way in which Max Contraction Training can increase your flexibility. As the muscles and joints are forced over time to contract against heavier weights in their strongest position of contraction, the ligaments will thicken from the compressive forces without undergoing undue shearing or stretching forces, such as those caused by full range (conventional) training practices. The increase in ligament thickness provides greater stability of the joints which reduces the need for secondary muscular support, and thus helps to produce a more flexible muscle.

In other words, Max Contraction Training will optimize your flexibility by bringing a greater degree of stability to your joints, which will afford you greater protection from injury.

If you still feel the need to warm up prior to your game, take a few easy practice swings. That—and Max Contraction Training—is all that is required.

10

MAX NUTRITION FOR PEAK PERFORMANCE AND WEIGHT CONTROL

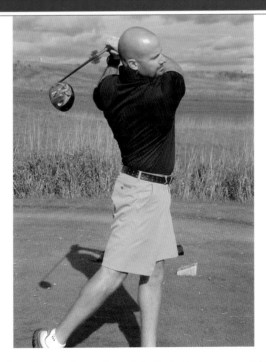

If muscles can be said to be the engines of the body, then proper nutrition is the fuel.

While training will make you stronger and stimulate lean tissue growth, that growth is produced during the recovery and over-compensation period that fall in between workouts. The body, however, does not accomplish this in a vacuum, it requires certain hormones, enzymes, and nutrients to build bigger, stronger muscle. And it is here that one must address the issue of nutrition.

Most golfers are overfat and over-nourished. In fact, most of the population are overfat and over-nourished. Indeed, it is the over-nourishment that produces the overfat condition. Without question, the most prevalent reason people give for joining Nautilus North (or any other fitness center) is a desire to lose fat. And while the desire to lose fat is nationwide, the fact remains that the majority of individuals seeking to lose fat fail in their task simply by not understanding the mechanism by which fat is lost, opting instead to try fad diets or partake of special herbs, minerals, and other supposedly "fat burning" supplements, or to perform aerobic exercises for several sessions a week. These people are often disappointed that, after a promising start, their fat loss goal seems further and further from their reach. Ultimately, most of these individuals will "fall off the wagon," giving up both the diet and the aerobics, and will end up fatter than they were before starting the regimen.

The reasons why such approaches typically end in failure are many, but two reasons stand out above all others. First, there is a difference between weight loss and fat loss, and anytime you cut back on macro-nutrients that your body needs (such as carbohydrates, fats, or proteins), then your diet is imbalanced, and the body and its tissues cannot survive without all of the nutrients that its survival entails. Consequently, you can only endure a diet in which a macronutrient is omitted for so long before the body rebels and you end up consuming more of the macro-nutrient than you did before.

In the case of low carbohydrate diets, which foolishly seem to come into vogue once every ten years or so (this fad is by no means new), it is true that one will lose a great deal of bodyweight quickly on carbohydrate restricted diets—but almost all of the weight lost is water, as each gram of glycogen stores with it three grams of water. As soon as dietary carbohydrate (the macronutrient that the body most readily converts to glucose) is removed, the body will utilize what glycogen is stored in the muscles and liver. Once this is used up, the body will then go to your muscle tissue to retrieve an amino acid (alinine), and send it to the liver to be converted into glucose, resulting in the body feeding on its own lean tissues in order to survive (not a good thing).

The primary reason for the body requiring carbohydrate in the diet is that the muscles, the brain, the central nervous system, and the peripheral nerves all derive 99.9 percent of the nutrition they need to survive from glucose (blood sugar), and carbohydrates are the energy source that the body most readily employs to create glucose.

Secondly, the reason that aerobic activities, per se, fail to strip much fat off the body is that one pound of fat can provide the body with sufficient fuel for up to ten hours of continuous aerobic activity, with the result that four to five sessions per week on a treadmill, in aerobics class, or on a stepping machine will make use of little more than an ounce or two of fat tissue for fuel. You can perform aerobics until you are quite literally blue in the face, and still not lose much in the way of body fat.

Strength training, by contrast, has actually been proven to be more effective than aerobics in reducing the levels of body fat in the body. Apart from the fat loss study I mentioned in Chapter Eight, in which "zero" conventional aerobic exercise was performed, Wayne Wescott, an exercise physiologist and strength-training consultant to the YMCA, also conducted a study in which he compared two groups of thirty-six men and women who had completed an eight-week program. All of them consumed a reduced caloric diet made up of 20 percent fat, 20 percent protein, and 60 percent carbohydrates. In addition, the subjects were required to exercise. One group combined a thirty-minute total body Nautilus strength training program with fifteen minutes of aerobic exercise. The other group did thirty minutes of aerobic activity only. The results were fascinating; the aerobics-only group lost an average of 3.2 pounds of fat, but the weight training/aerobic exercise group ended up losing an average of 10 pounds of fat—three times more fat loss than the aerobics-only group! It's significant to note that this group also gained two pounds of muscle per person, compared to a loss of a half a pound of muscle per person among the aerobics-only group (more on this shortly).

Another study conducted by researchers at Emory University in Atlanta revealed similar findings, this time with overweight women as their subjects. The women, who either did twenty minutes of aerobics three times a week or nothing at all, lost only 0.72 pounds of fat per pound of weight lost. Mary Ellen Sweeney, M.D., of the Emory Health Enhancement Program, reported that those who did twenty minutes of strength training retained more muscle mass—which translated into 85 percent of every pound they lost being fat tissue.

Muscle mass is the key. Let us suppose that, if you could add ten pounds of muscle to your body, each pound of new muscle will burn somewhere between 25 and 100 extra calories per day, thereby raising your metabolism by an extra 250 to 1,000 calories per day. As there are 3,500 calories in a pound of fat, the additional muscle mass will cause your body to turn to body fat for these extra calories at the cost of (in the higher scenario) two pounds of fat per week. Incidentally, this increase in your metabolism will continue even when you're not working out, so long as you have (and hold) that extra muscle tissue.

In truth, the reason why our metabolisms slow down with each passing decade of age is because we lose an estimated 6.6 pounds of muscle every decade once we exit our twenties, and with those 6.6 pounds of muscle, so, too, go the 165 to 660 calories a day they were causing our bodies to burn. If that muscle is put back on the body through strength training, then our metabolism correspondingly increases.

A Rational Approach to Fat Loss

The rational approach to fat loss is a scientific one: a straightforward combination of a properly conducted strength training program to gain (or re-gain) muscle mass, coupled with a well-balanced but calorie-reduced diet. It's based on the following fact:

Energy Intake (or Energy Output) = Weight Gain (or Weight Loss).

If, for instance, you take in more energy in the form of food than you use in a normal day's activities, then you will gain weight. If, on the other hand, you take in less than you use, you will lose weight. This translates to eating less (though it doesn't have to be a lot less) and expending sufficient energy to cause your body to build more muscle, which will then burn more calories while you are at rest. In order to make practical use of this advice, it is first necessary to be able to determine your body's actual caloric needs.

Basal metabolic rate

The body can be likened to an engine of sorts, and like most engines it needs fuel to operate. This fuel comes from the food we eat. What we put in our mouths is synthesized in a variety of complex chemical processes and is then used as fuel for basic biological work. This basic work—all the involuntary activity that keeps the machinery going—is called the basal metabolism. The speed at which this process operates for each individual is called the basal metabolic rate (or BMR). The BMR is the basic level of the body's daily energy needs—and these needs are substantial.

But the BMR is only part of the story. Our daily activities—from picking up a coffee cup to working out—also require energy. The energy that we use to sustain our BMR and our activity levels originates from calories. (For convenience, everyone uses the word "calorie" but food doesn't actually contain calories, it contains energy potential and it is this energy potential that is *measured* in calories; food supplies calories that are turned into energy or fuel for the body through a series of chemical transformations.) Your total calorie needs are based on your own personal BMR plus your daily energy needs for voluntary activity. It is essential to know this total if you are to control your weight. Here's a simple, accurate way to find your BMR and your total daily maintenance level:

If you're a man, add a zero to the end of your present weight and then add twice your weight. So, for example, if you weigh 150, your BMR would be 1,800 (150 with an extra 0 equals 1,500, plus twice 150, or 300, equals 1,800). If you're a woman, add a zero to the end of your weight and then add your weight (125 with an added 0 equals 1,250, plus 125 equals 1,375). Next, this figure must be adjusted for age since people tend to be less active after age twenty.

Adjust the BMR for age by subtracting 2 percent for each decade of age. If you're thirty, subtract 6 percent; if you're forty, 8 percent, and so on. Using these examples, the 150-pound, thirty-year-old man would have an adjusted BMR of 1,692 (1,800 minus 6 percent [108] equals 1,692). The woman's BMR at thirty would be 1,293 (1,375 minus 6 percent [82] equals 1,293). The body's energy balance is remarkably precise, so it is important to be exactly careful about energy intake as you age. If, as you grow older, you burn less energy by, say, a 150 calories a day, but continue to eat in the same way you did when you burning that extra 150 calories, you'll gain more than a pound of fat a month.

Once you have determined your BMR, you should make an addition to this that will reflect the cost in calories you require for your daily voluntary movement. Remember this activity can range from very heavy physical exertion (athletes in training, manual labor, climbing) to very light work, (sitting in front of a computer terminal all day, driving). But on the average, unless you're extremely active or passive, this rate of consumption can be figured at 30 percent of the age-adjusted BMR. So once again, taking the 150-pound man as an example, his total daily need will be 2,200 (BMR 1,692 + 30 percent or 508 = 2,200). The 125-pound woman's rate will be 1,681 (BMR 1,293 + 30 percent or 388 = 1,681). Since these calorie counting and BMR figures are not absolutely exact (for precision, one had better go to a body composition center such as Body Comp), it's easier to round off the final figure to the nearest zero. (Some nutritionists suggest using an overall figure of 17.5 calories per pound of body weight per day for men and 15.5 for women. However, this will give you a slightly higher total. You may want to begin your weight control program using this formula.)

3,500 calories

This number—3,500—is the absolute key to weight control. It represents the number of calories in a pound of fat. You can forget everything else you've ever read about dieting. From this point on, 3,500 is the bottom line.

Going back to the simple arithmetic of weight loss (Energy Intake or Energy Expenditure = Weight Gain or Loss), it's easy to see that you have to consume 3,500 extra calories, over and above your daily needs (BMR plus energy expenditure), to gain a pound of body fat and you have to cut your consumption by 3,500 calories to lose a pound of body fat. How much is 3,500 calories? It's:

- 10 cups of spaghetti and meatballs
- 10 cups of chili with beans

- 17 seventeen waffles without syrup and butter
- 35 doughnuts
- 1 whole pecan pie

In other words, it's a lot. In fact, 3,500 calories is far more than most of us eat in an entire day. If you regularly consume 2,500 calories a day and maintain your weight, you'd have to eat five doughnuts a day or two and a half waffles a day for a week to compile the extra 3,500 calories needed to add a pound of fat. With this in mind, it's easier to see why large, permanent weight losses (or gains, for that matter) are impossible in a short period of time. Let's say your daily needs total 2,500 calories. Obviously, at that rate of consumption, if you ate nothing at all you couldn't lose a pound of fat a day, and you'd have to eat a hefty 6,000 calories to gain a pound a day.

To lose weight you need to cut back your total daily calorie intake but you don't have to cut that much. If you continue to eat a variety of foods sensibly (essentially your current diet) and cut back from 2,500 calories to 2,000 per day—a reduction of only 500—you could lose a pound a week (500 per day × 7 days = 3,500). Not bad, and not that difficult either. At that modest rate, in seventy days, you could lose ten pounds and keep it off because the loss was accomplished slowly and painlessly without really depriving yourself of anything.

Now, if you *combine* this reduction in calories with the additional energy expenditure required by the Max Contraction exercises, you can increase the speed of weight loss because you'll be increasing your calorie deficit. A reduction of 500 calories per day plus an energy expenditure of approximately 250 calories once a week when you work out, plus the additional muscle you will be building could see you with a total of 3,750 calories a week and result in the loss of slightly more than two additional pounds of fat in two weeks. That doesn't sound like much, but viewed over six months, that's a loss of over twelve pounds of pure body fat, which could transform the way you look.

It sounds easy—and it is easy—if you can discipline yourself and stay with it. At best, the ability of human beings to regulate their food intake is very poor, and sedentary people almost always eat more than they need. And exercise is important to weight control—the right type of exercise, that is—as it tends to decrease appetite, and the rise in body temperature that occurs during exercise also inhibits hunger. Physiologists and nutritionists agree that the intensity of the exercise is also important in calorie cost, and only muscular work, in whatever form, uses the body's energy. Sitting and thinking about exercise won't do a thing but help broaden your behind.

Since calories count so highly, here's how I would suggest you keep track. Before you begin the program, weigh yourself (an ordinary bathroom scale will do but use the same scale each time), and buy an inexpensive calorie-counting book and a pocket-sized note pad. For the next five days eat your normal diet, but record everything you eat, and I mean everything. Don't forget that piece of chewing gum or the milk in your coffee. Every time you pop something in your mouth write it down along with the quantity. At the end of each day, use the calorie counter and total the calories consumed. If you've been a faithful recorder, you'll probably be surprised and shocked at the sheer number of entries. Most people eat much more (and much more often) than they think they do. At the end of five days, add the daily figures and divide by five. This will give you a daily average. Now weigh yourself a second time. You may have gained or lost a pound but if you have continued to eat the way you normally do, you should have remained at about the same weight as when you started counting. This means the calorie figure you have in your hand is your maintenance level of caloric intake. If you didn't gain or lose, it also represents your total daily needs at your current weight.

Reduce your calorie intake, add exercise, and watch your weight go down and stay down. For the first few weeks I'd advise you to continue to keep a daily calorie count. It's a good incentive. You'll soon know the calories of most items so you won't have to keep referring to the book and you'll begin to make those trade-offs that make it possible to hit your daily target, but with a variety of foods. For total nutrition your diet must be well balanced.

The well-balanced diet

It may be simplistic to say that the well-balanced diet is "a little bit of everything," but in fact, that's exactly what it is. Nutritionists have divided foods into six groups based on similarities in nutritive value and their role in the diet. A well-balanced diet includes several servings from each group every day. Here's how they break down:

1. Meat, poultry, dry beans, and nuts group: Two to three servings of meat, fish, poultry, or eggs. Nuts and beans can be substituted. (Note: A serving size is average (i.e., three ounces of meat) and does not include gravies or sauces. The grains should not be included in cakes, pies, or other sweets. This does not mean that you shouldn't have gravy on your potatoes or cake for dessert, just that such items generally add only calories and little of nutritive value.)
2. Vegetables: Three to five servings.
3. Fruits: Two to four servings.
4. Milk, yogurt, and cheese group: Two to three servings of milk or servings of cheese, butter, or ice cream.
5. Breads and cereals: Four or more servings.
6. Fats, oils, and sweets: Use sparingly.

There is also a "seventh category"—snacks—but it's inconsequential and unnecessary if you're well looked after in the first six groups and highly undesirable if your goal is to lose body fat. The six groups are not the be-all and end-all of eating and nutrition, but they are a reliable guide to well-balanced consumption. They are analyzed in much greater detail in books devoted to nutrition (not diet books) and individual adjustments can be made to suit your basic needs, your additional needs for energy consumption (exercise and pregnancy can increase the total amount of food you eat and consequently the nutrients you ingest), products available in your part of the country, and your lifestyle.

A person who eats a diet that includes most of the foods in these six groups each day should not need vitamin or mineral supplements of any kind. The nutrients provided in the well-balanced diet include:

Macronutrients

There are four macronutrients—carbohydrates, fats, proteins, and water. They are the body's only important sources of energy and they are therefore used in great quantities. The carbohydrates, much maligned by the diet doctors, are the body's main source of fuel. They're stored in the muscles and liver in the form of energy-giving glycogen. Fats, stored in the muscles, under the skin, and around body organs, are the second-best source of energy. Protein, though it enjoys the best publicity, is a poor energy provider at any time, and the body has no way of storing it. Water may be the most important of all the nutrients. We can live for some time without protein, fat, and carbohydrate, but we only last a few days without water. Let's take a closer look:

Carbohydrates   Carbohydrates are chemical compounds of sugar, starches, and cellulose (fiber) containing carbon, hydrogen, and oxygen. The most important carbohydrate is glucose, the body's primary energy source. The sugar molecules in food are called monosaccharides (individual molecules), disaccharides (pairs), and polysaccharides (three or more). The body can only absorb monosaccharides so it chemically breaks down di- and polysaccharides into the usable form. Glucose, fructose, and galactose are the only monosaccharides that find their way to the liver, where fructose and galactose are converted to glucose and used for energy. Sugar, because it contains readily usable glucose, is absorbed into the bloodstream very quickly. Starches need to be broken down and are absorbed more slowly.

Interestingly, the original source of the glucose doesn't matter in the slightest. Glucose is glucose whether it comes from an ice cream soda or mashed potatoes. As a source of energy, however, pure sugar or honey are poor choices; they are absorbed immediately and may give a "rush" of energy, but there is no lasting effect. The more complex carbohydrates found in such starches as potatoes and peas take longer for the body to process and provide a longer-lasting energy source.

Ordinarily, there is less than a quarter of an ounce of glucose available in the bloodstream at any one time. But the body has ten to twelve ounces more in storage in the heart and muscle tissue. This reserve energy is used during prolonged exercise. Roughly 50 percent of the daily calorie intake should consist of carbohydrates.

Fats   Fats, or lipids, are chemical compounds that don't dissolve in water. Most fats (about 98 percent) are called triglycerides, of which some are saturated and come from animals and some are unsaturated and come from plants. Fats are very caloric—about 3,500 calories per pound, as you'll recall. This is more than twice the calorie density of carbohydrates. Low-fat diets are very effective for trimming the pounds, but much of the fat consumed daily is hidden (in meat, milk, cheese, and nuts) and difficult to eliminate without excluding other valuable nutrients as well. Fat should make up less than 35 percent of your daily diet, especially if you're concerned about the potentially damaging effects cholesterol may have on the cardiovascular system.

Protein   Protein is the organic material that, next to water, is the primary structural material of the body's cells and tissues. There are about twenty amino acids in protein and at least nine of these (the "essential" amino acids) have to come from the daily diet. But just as the body doesn't care where it gets its glucose, it isn't concerned about the source of its protein. In other words, beans are as good as meat.

Nutritionist Ronald Deutsch feels that "protein has become the dietary lure to which the consumer consistently rises, like a hungry trout on a quiet morning." There is truth in what he says. It's a fact, of course, that protein is absolutely essential for growth and repair of the body's tissues, but it has yet to be proven that more than enough of any essential element of nutrition is better than merely enough.

The average adult needs about seventy grams of protein per day for normal growth and development. This translates to about nine ounces of broiled hamburger, which also contain about thirty grams of fat. Yet I know bodybuilders who eat 500 grams of protein a day thinking it will help them gain additional muscle. The protein they're eating obviously contains calories just as fats and carbohydrates do. The extra protein doesn't help. In fact, it hurts, because the excess is stored as fat, even when the extra protein comes from steak. You'd need to eat a little more than five pounds of steak to get the 500 grams of protein. Unfortunately, this amount of meat contains more than 8,000 calories and about 675 grams of fat. Think of the exercise necessary to work off those extra calories. I'd estimate it at more than fifteen hours of intense work. With the cost of meat what it is, this type of useless excess is expensive in more ways than one; if your daily diet consists of 15 percent protein, you have nothing to worry about.

Water   Water is obviously important when you consider that the body is 60 percent water. Water not only contains valuable minerals but also it acts as a lubricant, a shock absorber between cells, a digestion aid, and is the body's principal means of cooling, performing the essential job of maintaining the body's normal temperature.

In the course of an average day the body loses water steadily, though much of this loss (about 50 percent) is unseen. On a hot day it's not uncommon to lose five to eight quarts of fluid, which, of course, must be replaced either by drinking liquids (again, it doesn't matter what you drink—with the exception of alcohol—nor does the temperature of the drink matter) or through the food normally consumed. A surprising amount of seemingly solid food contains a high percentage of water. Meats can be as much as half water while most fruits and vegetables are at least 70 percent water.

If you get thirsty while exercising, don't hesitate to drink fluids. Your body is trying to tell you something. The idea that the athlete shouldn't drink while practicing has been discarded. Drinking fluids during exercise does not cause cramps—an old but persistent error. Remember though, immediate weight-loss during exercise is almost all fluid. Exercise eventually cuts into the fat content of your body but it takes time for this effect to appear.

Micronutrients

Vitamins   Vitamins are organic substances that play a major role in the control of the body's metabolic processes. They help to process the macronutrients—carbohydrates, fats, and protein—and serve as aids to the body's own self-produced enzymes (forming coenzymes), which function as biochemical catalysts.

The body cannot manufacture its own vitamins so they must be obtained from the diet. This is not at all difficult if you're eating a well-balanced diet because the daily vitamin requirement is one-eighth of a teaspoon. Interestingly, though nutritionists agree that vitamins are essential to good health, there is little agreement on which vitamins (if any) are most important, the proper dosage, or who needs them.

It does seem clear, however, that vitamins in any amount do not cure disease or provide extra health protection. Ronald Deutsch says, "In extra doses, used essentially as medicines, vitamins and minerals cure scarcely anything except deficiencies in vitamins and minerals." This, of course, includes the extravagant claims made for vitamin C (as a cold cure) and vitamin E (as a hedge against aging). Deutsch's views are underlined in a report by the American Psychiatric Association which concludes, "The results and claims of the advocates of megavitamin therapy have not been confirmed." The APA panel found "the massive publicity which they [megavitamin therapists] promulgate via radio, the lay press and popular books . . . to be deplorable."

It is possible that vegetarians, food faddists, people on low-calorie diets, and very fussy eaters may not get the United States Recommended Daily Allowance of vitamins. But even this is unlikely (and easily rectified with a multivitamin supplement) because the fat-soluble vitamins—A, D, E, and K—are stored in the body's fat and don't need to be consumed daily. The water-soluble vitamins—C and eight B vitamins—should be consumed daily but they are very easy to acquire even in a moderately well-balanced diet. One other point—vitamins do not provide energy and there is absolutely no need to increase your vitamin intake even during heavy exercise.

Minerals   Minerals are chemicals found in the soil and passed to humans through plants and animals. They are vital to life processes but only in small quantities. They activate hormones, prevent anemia, and are essential in controlling heartbeat and muscle contraction. The most important, or at least those minerals needed in the largest amounts, are sodium, magnesium, calcium, and potassium. Other minerals, including iron, cobalt, and iodine, are needed in trace amounts. (See chart elsewhere in this chapter.) Most minerals can be obtained from the daily diet if that diet includes vegetables, fruits, grains, and dairy products.

Diets and Why They Work

Most diets work in the short run because, whatever they may promise about eating all you want, their main trick is to get you to eat less.

The big "secret" is a reduction in your caloric consumption, often by excluding one of the macronutrients, usually carbohydrates (bread, potatoes, pasta, desserts). Psychologically, most such diets quickly become boring and you tend to eat even less than the diet's suggested allowance. What the Stillman, Atkins, and most other diets do is reduce the carbohydrate intake to below sixty grams a day. This causes weight loss. Here's why: carbohydrates are the body's main source of energy. The low-carbohydrate diet forces the body to reach into itself for substitute forms of fuel—some of its protein and stored fat. This shift in internal chemical processes results in more waste products. These wastes activate the kidneys and they, in turn, respond by getting rid of the waste. This reduces the body's water content. This loss can conceivably add up to ten pounds in a week—but it's almost all fluid. Since fat contains very little water, you aren't losing fat.

Nutritional scientist Ronald Deutsch puts the problem in perspective in his book *Realities of Nutrition*. Deutsch says, "to give some idea of how much stored energy fat represents, consider the 'typical' young American woman, at five feet, five inches, and 128 pounds. A little over 25 of those pounds are in fat. And this much fat has enough energy potential to meet all the woman's needs for about 45 days, if she gets no food at all."

Your body has a tremendous amount of energy in reserve even if you aren't overweight. It obviously takes a severe and prolonged energy shortage to make any progress against excess fat.

What Is Overweight?

As I've said, you can't be overweight by even a few pounds and be totally fit because that few pounds is excess fat. The body has a sophisticated system of storing fuel for later use—keeping the tank filled. That extra fuel, over and above the combined BMR/Energy Expenditure rate, is converted to fat (the few pounds mentioned above). The body is designed to store a certain amount of fat for energy reserve (it's an extremely compact fuel supply providing twice as much energy per calorie as either protein or carbohydrate), for insulation, for padding, and for the lean times. But these days, in this country at least, there are relatively few lean times, so most of us store fat, fat, and more fat.

This excess serves no useful purpose, it's potentially harmful, and it's certainly unsightly. It's what makes us overweight.

There are a number of different tables that give recommended weight ranges adjusted to height. These charts aren't of much value except to show the wide range of human variation. They don't take into consideration such individual differences as body composition (muscle weighs more than fat), skeletal size, and body type (ectomorph, mesomorph, or endomorph), all of which have an influence on weight.

The charts give arbitrary numbers and should be used only with that fact in mind, but, with or without a chart, you can tell if you're overweight. Subjectively, you know if you feel overweight and you can confirm your worst fears by looking at yourself in the mirror. Objectively, you can tell if your clothes are getting too tight and you can use the scale. If you fall outside the upper ranges of any of the height-weight charts, you are overweight.

If you are 20 percent above the recommended weight on the charts, you are probably not just overweight, but obese, a dreaded word in our society. No matter how little your food intake exceeds your energy output, you're going to put on weight. When this imbalance goes on for a time, you get overweight; if it continues, you get badly overweight; and finally, if you don't put a stop to it, you become obese.

There is evidence to indicate that obesity can also result from too little physical activity as well as just overeating. One study, using pedometers, showed that non-obese subjects were twice as active as those who were obese. And factors such as heredity, body type, stress, and anxiety can also be causes of overweight and eventual obesity.

No matter the causes, if you are heavier than your "ideal" weight (usually your weight at age twenty), you are overweight. If you are 20 percent above that weight you are obese, unless you're very muscular; and if you're 25 percent over, you are subjecting yourself to potential health problems, not the least of which is heart disease.

If you can't remember your weight at twenty (or if you were overweight then), and you can't honestly tell by looking in the mirror, then the "pinch test" is a good measure of fatness. The fat deposits under the skin (basically) reflect the total fat stored throughout the body. One of the best places to pinch is the back of the arm right behind the triceps. It's a little hard to take this measurement by yourself so you may want to ask a friend to help. With your arm hanging straight down, take hold of the skin with your thumb and forefinger at the midpoint between the elbow and the shoulder. Pull the pinched area away from the muscle. The fat will pull away with skin. If you're a man under thirty the layer of fat and skin pinched away should measure less than six-tenths of an inch; for a woman, less than 1.1 inches. If you're a man over thirty, the fold should be less than nine-tenths of an inch and for a woman, less than 1.25 inches. If the measurement is greater than it should be, you can consider yourself overweight. But don't let this scare you. It's something you need to know.

Body Composition

About 60 percent of body weight in men and 50 percent in women is water. Men have about 12 percent body fat on the average and women about 25 percent. The rest of the body (about 25 percent) is muscle, bone, blood, tissues, and organs, or "lean body mass." Muscle is heavier than fat and contains much more water (about 70 percent compared to 15 percent). Since fat contains little water, the percent of total water in an obese person is lower than in a non-obese person. The relation between total water and fat-free body weight (lean body mass) should remain constant, so when you're overweight, body composition is distorted. A combination of diet and exercise will result in the loss of fat (a large proportion of body weight), the addition of muscle, and is a very effective method of restoring the body's composition and shape.

Intensive physical training using progressive resistance machines will increase muscle mass and reduce the body's fat content. How? First, exercise with weights increases skeletal muscle size and this muscle displaces fatty tissue throughout the body. Second, strength training increases the capacity of the body's oxygen-transporting system through the cardiovascular training effect attained by the intensity of the exercise routine. It is a physiological fact that the greater the ability of the system to utilize oxygen, the greater the ability to use fat as fuel. Training increases the oxygen supply to the muscle cells so that exercise is largely performed aerobically with less lactic acid build-up. A low oxygen supply to the working muscle limits the usable fuel to carbohydrates. The less fit person produces more lactic acid which inhibits the use of fat as fuel. Conscientious weight control, along with exercise, also serves to maintain the correct balance of water and fat to muscle, bone, and other tissues.

Diet for the Golfer

Bodybuilding champion Mike Mentzer once told me of a friend of his, a competitive bodybuilder, who was so brainwashed by the health-food industry that he downed a special protein drink every two hours every day. If he didn't have this glass of magic elixir he actually got a headache and within a couple of days his ability to lift weights would decrease because he believed he was losing the protein his muscles required for strength and growth.

Bodybuilders have to be the worst offenders when it comes to believing in the magic power of foods and diet. The magic food or super pill may result in exceptional gains, provided, of course, that the bodybuilder's diet is adequate in every other way. In other words, if you're not eating right, nothing will help, and even if you are eating well, the special items are only placebos. The effects are in your head, not your body.

Of course this is nothing new. Athletes have been fanatics for centuries. The first recorded attempt to influence performance through diet occurred in Greece more than 2,500 years ago. Two athletes switched from the basic vegetarian diet of the time to a meat diet, thinking that something in the meat would replace the suspected loss of muscle during heavy workouts—just like my friend. Yet all the research done in this field is summed up by nutritionist Jean Mayer: "The concept that any well-balanced diet is all that athletes actually require for peak performance has not been superseded."

Even for competitive athletes there is no substitute for a well-balanced diet. Immediately before competition some athletes tend to eat more, but the increased energy expenditure in preparing for the events more than offsets the increased energy consumption. Research also has shown that greatly reduced or greatly increased protein consumption has no effect whatever on performance.

If a golfer is over-nourished or even adequately well nourished and yet he's not making progress, it stands to reason that his "problem" is not nutritional. If you're "over-nourished," then, by definition, you've more than covered all of your nutritional bases—so how can nutrition be a problem? If you're over-nourished or well nourished, and you aren't progressing, then your problem can only be related to training and recovery. In fact—and this is the key point—training is the first requirement, adequate rest and recovery is the second—and only then, in a distant third place, does nutrition enter the picture. And when it does factor in, it does so quite simply—all that is required in the way of nutrition for golfers is to consume a well-balanced diet, which I've already gone into some detail about. A well-balanced diet, by definition, provides the body with all the nutrients it needs. However, golfers have been subjected to thousands of pages worth of propaganda put out by the supplement companies through the various magazines over the years and thus have concluded that they *need* to supplement their diets in order to create more energy or achieve peak performance. Supplements do not build anything quicker. In fact, if you take the time to examine the small print on most supplement labels you will read the following: As with all supplements, use of this product will not promote faster or greater muscular gains. This product is however, a nutritious low-fat food supplement which, like other foods, provides nutritional support for weight training athletes.

Nutritional supplements, it should be pointed out, were developed not by golfers or for golfers but by medical researchers to provide, in fact, "supplementation" to people who through genetic or other health problems were unable to overcome nutritional deficiencies; they were never intended to be used by healthy individuals consuming well balanced diets, because medical and nutritional scientists understand what I've just revealed—that a healthy individual consuming a well balanced diet, by definition, is getting everything he needs—and the human body does not utilize nutrients beyond *need*.

Still, despite the foregoing facts, many golfers continue to feel that they require a super-abundance—and certainly more than a balanced diet would allot—of the various vitamins, minerals, and other supplements. However, I will tell you categorically that this is simply not true.

And for proof of this you need look no further than the golfing and/or fitness magazines of ten years back. For instance, if you pick up a copy of *Muscle Builder* or *Power* from the 1970s you'll read that it was milk and egg protein powder; in the 1980s it was amino acids that were *de rigeur*; in the 1990s it was MET-Rx. Presently it's creatine phosphate. In ten years, it will be something else. How scientific.

With each passing decade, the "must have" supplements from the previous decade drop from sight—so how "must have" were they? In the 1960s, for example, it was vitamin E capsules, which were being touted as wonder pills that would protect you from everything from smog and heart attacks to sexual problems. It was not uncommon then for their manufacturers to recommend up to 500 units of the vitamin E to be taken after each meal. But what is the truth about how much "E" you really need to ingest on a daily basis? For this answer, we can't look to the vitamin E supplement salesmen, but rather to independent bodies such as the Food and Nutrition Board. Going back to our example about vitamin E, we note that the RDA for this vitamin is fifteen international units daily. Thus, the "1,500 units a day" supplement (500 after each meal) actually supplies over three months worth of the RDA for this one vitamin. But ask yourself: "Is it likely that the RDA Committee is grossly in error about the amount of vitamin E needed for optimum health?" Or, putting a sharper point on it, consider the fact that our species was only able to survive and evolve by eating food that it could readily obtain. Do you honestly think that there should exist large natural barriers to our ability to access the foods needed for the maintenance of our health? I mean, it's simple common sense—to obtain the "recommended" dosage of 1,500 I.U.s of vitamin E each day our ancestors would have had to look for foods rich in "E" such as nuts, almonds being one of the best sources. To get this amount of vitamin E would require eighteen pounds of almonds a day. And wheat germ, which has also received much press as an excellent source of vitamin E, would require you to consume twenty-seven pounds of it a day in order to obtain 1,500 I.U.s. This is an extraordinary amount of food! Just one tablespoon of wheat germ weighs six grams and provides twenty-three calories. Simple mathematics reveals that twenty-seven pounds of wheat germ would require over 2,000 tablespoons a day! Which, in turn, would contain over 46,000 calories. Think about this. Is it really realistic to believe that a person can't obtain good health without either supplements or twenty-seven pounds of wheat germ? Don't be a health food fanatic—be a golfer. They're two different things.

The supplement companies respond that what the Senate Subcommittee on Nutrition recommends—the Recommended Dietary Allowances or RDAs—just aren't set high enough for good health and that the food we eat is sorely lacking in nutrients due to over-processing. Therefore, they argue, we need to supplement our diet. The truth is that the RDAs are estimated to *exceed* the requirements of most individuals, which would thereby ensure that the needs of nearly all are met. I suppose a possible exception to this rule might be in the RDA estimates of calories, or energy—but even here, obviously, it would not be a good idea to set a generous excess, since obesity is a widespread problem. The Board, for those who don't know, was assembled under the auspices of the National Academy of Science's National Research Council and is composed of large numbers of America's more respected nutritional scientists. Moreover, its membership changes periodically, both to share the burden of the work and to broaden the variety of legitimately informed opinions. The Board's Committee on Dietary Allowances is composed of subcommittees for each nutrient, or in some cases, for groups of nutrients. And it is the job of the scientists on these subcommittees to constantly reassess what is known of the nutrients, and keep up to date on the latest research reports. They also study the quantities of nutrients in the American food supply, their effects on the body, and any additional relevant information about the public's health and eating habits. Just about every five years, the Committee on Dietary Allowances publishes an updated report called *Recommended Dietary Allowances* (RDAs). This report sets out guideline recommendations for different population groups, according to height, sex, age, and weight. Thus a Recommended Dietary Allowance (RDA) for seventeen different groups of people is estimated for every nutrient about which there is sufficient data to make an informed judgment. A misperception has arisen over the years—largely promulgated by supplement companies—that the RDAs are minimums for survival, whereas in fact, they are set up to include generous safety margins. RDAs, under different names, are also set in other countries, such as Canada and Great Britain, and by United Nations agencies, and these are usually lower than the American RDAs for several nutrients. In practical terms, these committees make recommendations which should provide an excess of any given nutrient for at least 95 percent of people. Even this is very conservatively estimated, however. For example, back in their 1968 report the Committee's RDA for vitamin C for the average adult male was estimated to be sixty milligrams a day. In 1974, based on revised information, the Committee lowered this recommendation to forty-five milligrams a day—so by and large the RDAs are, if anything, overly generous, rather than inadequate. I go into the whole issue of

No supplement is going to turn a duffer into a scratch golfer.

nutrition and supplement fraud in my book *Max Contraction Training* in much greater detail. For now, let these few words serve as a reminder of the deceptions that abound in the world of golf regarding the issue of nutrition for peak performance. The supplement industry is reportedly an $18 billion a year business, which buys a lot of lobby power and a lot of advertising. If you're one of those golfers who have been supporting this deception by purchasing such supplements, stop wasting your money on these useless supplements and get on a Max Contraction Training schedule and a well-balanced diet. If you train hard, eat a well-balanced diet, and get adequate rest, you will be doing all that you can to improve your golf game.

11
SENIOR
BENEFITS

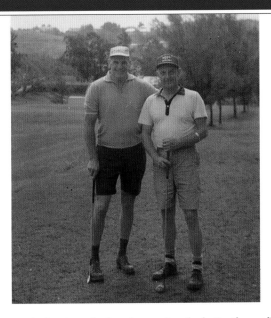

The longer one can retain the strength of one's muscles, the better the quality of life one will enjoy—and the longer they can enjoy playing the game of golf. Here, NHL hockey legend Syl Apps (left) and former track and field star Bill Little (right) take advantage of their enhanced fitness levels on the course (both were in their mid 60s when this photo was taken).

Many senior citizens shy away from strength training—to their detriment. I'm at a loss to explain why this is so, given that there is so much data in favor of their lifting weights. Perhaps some are from an era when strength training simply wasn't done, and most certainly not a part of one's weekly routine. Others might suffer the needless fear that resistance training is a dangerous activity for those over the age of sixteen, or falsely believe that it is solely the domain of football players, bodybuilders, and Olympic weightlifters. Or maybe it's that they are simply unaware of the data. If so, then this chapter will provide them, as it is the senior population that probably has the most to gain from a proper resistance training program such as Max Contraction.

A recent study conducted by physiologist Wayne Wescott to determine the benefits of a brief resistance training program on the body composition, muscle strength, joint flexibility, and functional ability of nineteen non-ambulatory senior citizens revealed some very encouraging news. Over a span of fourteen weeks, training but twice a week for six minutes a workout, performing one set of each of six different exercises, doctors found that the senior residents of John Knox Village Campus (which includes the Med Center, Assisted Living, and Independent Living facilities) in Orange City, Florida, the average age of which was 88.5 years, were able to dramatically improve their body composition, their muscle strength, their joint flexibility, functional capacity and mobility.

Many of the seniors who started the study confined to a wheelchair were able to walk without its aid at the study's conclusion. The nineteen subjects who completed the fourteen-week strength training program reported that it was a positive experience and planned to continue their exercise sessions. According to the lead trainer, patients liked the challenge of serious strength training and saw much more improvement than when on a program of resistance exercise with light cuff weights. The researchers concluded that in addition to the benefits to our senior population, such programs should be instrumental in reducing health care costs, thereby benefiting society in general.

Actually Reversing Aging

McMaster University published a study that revealed that strength training for people sixty-five and older can actually *reverse* important aging effects on skeletal muscles to the point where they work like those found in people four decades younger.

The study was supported by the U.S. National Institute of Health, and looked at DNA expression in the muscle cells of twenty-five healthy seniors who had undergone twice-weekly resistance training for six months. It concentrated in particular on the cellular mitochondria, the "powerhouses" that fuel activity in cells. They are typically depleted in older people, with many of the genes that affect them turned on or off by age. This depletion results in a loss of muscle mass and many of the mobility restrictions often found in seniors. The lead researcher in the study, a man named Tarnopolsky, said that the genetic "fingerprints" of exercising seniors actually shifted from their age-altered state to one more closely resembling those found in young men and women in their mid twenties to thirties. "We improved or reversed to a large extent the gene signature of aging," he said. This reversal was accompanied by a 50 percent improvement in strength among seniors. He went on to state that weight training might remove some of the mitochondria damaged by age-related stresses, replacing them with genetically intact ones. As well, it may turn on genes, switched off by age, that offer muscle cells protection from damage. The seniors in the study, who had an average age of seventy, had no diseases that affected their mitochondrial function and had never participated in weight training before.

More benefits

Researchers have discovered that many of the degenerative diseases and most of the general weakness that accompanies the aging process are related to loss of muscle mass and strength. Although a certain amount of strength loss is inevitable, numerous studies—too many to be ignored—have shown that senior adults can maintain and regain muscle mass and strength at any age. Postmenopausal women, older men, and even those well into their nineties have all improved their muscular and skeleton structure and function through relatively simple programs of strength training.

The research results are remarkable: strength exercise has produced improved muscular fitness, increased bone mineral density, enhanced gastrointestinal transit, resulted in greater glucose utilization, better balance, reduced low back pain, and decreased arthritic discomfort and higher levels of self confidence and independence.

How often?

A study published by the *Journal of the American Geriatrics Society* in 1999 (47 [10]:1208–14) indicated that such gains could be obtained with only *one* workout a week—and more studies support this. A second comparison of once-weekly and twice-weekly strength training in older adults conducted by the Academic Health Care Center of the New York College of Osteopathic Medicine and the Department of Physical Therapy, at the New York Institute of Technology, School of Health Professions, Behavioral and Life Sciences, concluded that one set of exercises performed once weekly to the point of muscle fatigue improved strength as well as twice-weekly exercises in the older adult.

We have conducted our own research over the past three years at Nautilus North, most of which has been published, and we've seen incredible results from as little as two minutes of strength training performed once every seven to ten days. Results such as significant reductions in blood pressure and cholesterol levels, diabetics being able to reduce their nightly insulin intake by up to 70 percent, and strength and mobility improving from having to get around with two canes and only being able to leg press 60 pounds, to not needing canes and being able to leg press in excess of 800 pounds!

How high is up?

Doug McGuff, M.D., who owns and operates Ultimate Exercise in South Carolina (www.ultimate-exercise.com) has a client that trains once a week with three exercises and has been doing so for seven years. This man performs a pulling exercise (seated row) with 280 pounds, bench presses 320 pounds and leg presses 600 pounds—and he's ninety-three years old!

The Anti-Aging Prescription

There are ten bio-markers of aging:

1. Bone density: Because calcium tends to be lost from the bones when people age, it makes the skeleton weaker, less dense and more brittle, which typically leads to osteoporosis.

2. Body temperature regulation: The body is supposed to maintain an internal temperature of 98.6 degrees, but as people grow older they tend to lose muscle and the heat that muscle provides, thus becoming more vulnerable in their body temperature to hot and cold, which often leads to illness.

3. Basal metabolic rate: Our rate of energizing or determining how many calories our bodies require to sustain their internal processes, declines by 2 percent per decade after the age of twenty.

4. Blood sugar tolerance: The body's ability to use glucose in the blood stream declines with age, thereby raising the risk for type 2 diabetes, which is one of the fastest growing spreading diseases in the country.

5. A decline in muscle strength: Older people are less strong because of the gradual deterioration of the muscles and motor nerves, which begins at the age of thirty for most people.

6. The fat content of the body: Between the ages of twenty and sixty-five, the average person doubles his ratio of fat to muscle. This process is exacerbated by a sedentary lifestyle and over eating. Exercise can often serve to retard appetite and, conversely, when you're not training, you tend to be more hungry—and to eat more often.

7. Aerobic capacity: By the age of sixty-five the body's ability to use oxygen efficiently declines by 30 to 40 percent.

8. Cholesterol and HDL ratios: Around age fifty HDL (or "High Density Lipoproteins," the so-called "good" cholesterol that protects the body against heart disease) loses ground to the LDL (or "Low Density Lipoproteins," the so-called "bad" cholesterol); a phenomenon that dramatically increases the risk of heart attack.

9. A decline in muscle mass: The average American loses 6.6 pounds of muscle with each decade after young adulthood and the rate of loss increases after the age of forty-five (but only if you don't do anything to replace it).

10. Blood pressure: The majority of Americans show a steady increase of blood pressure with each decade of age.

And the one and only activity that's been proven scientifically to affect all ten of these bio-markers of aging is strength training. No other activity comes close not even aerobics! And Max Contraction is the most efficient form of strength training available.

If you're a senior citizen and you haven't strength trained—start. Your quality of life will increase enormously.

12
QUESTIONS AND ANSWERS

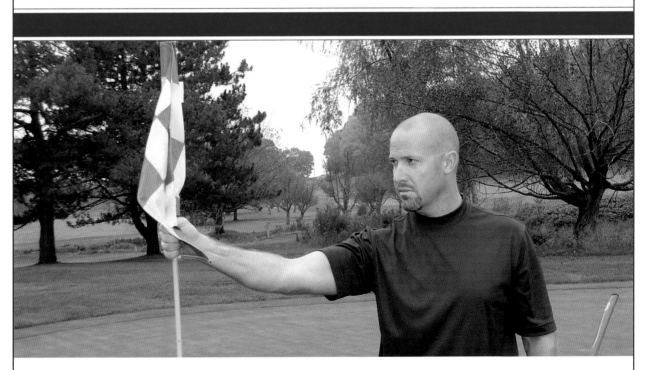

Proper strength training yields benefits that will serve you well throughout your life—both on and off the course.

Q: I understand what you're saying about training. I'm just curious, though, how does Tiger Woods train?

A: That's a good question. Ron Kaspriske, who writes for *Golf Digest*, has written an online article (August 2004) about Woods's strength training sessions:

> When he is not competing, Woods typically spends three or four hours a day, five times a week, in the gym. For these high-intensity workouts, said my source (let's call him Deep Bunker), he varies the focus of each session from strength training to improvements in cardiovascular performance. He usually starts with 30 minutes of some kind of cardiovascular warm-up exercise such as pedaling on a stationary bike. Then he'll perform a 30-minute session of total-body stretching, focusing on the muscles of the legs and trunk. A trainer assists him with physical therapy, manipulating his body to prepare the joints for the rigors of swinging a golf club as violently as Woods does. Everything from the kneecaps to the vertebrae are prepared for battle.

If the above information is true, then it is little wonder that Tiger has been inconsistent as of late—he is grossly overtrained. Whatever gains he presently enjoys, he would have achieved sooner or he might even have progressed further (i.e., become stronger) had he allowed his body the time it required to build the strength and size his workouts might have stimulated. However, since hard work and long work are mutually exclusive, Tiger isn't training hard enough to stimulate much in the way of gains as hard training would leave him physically unable to work out for "three to four hours a day, five times a week." That's fifteen to twenty hours a week, folks—in the gym. This represents nothing more than a wealthy man who is a mark for personal fitness trainers who get paid by the hour. Such a program produces considerable wear and tear stresses on the body and allows virtually no time off to allow the body to recoup the energy expended and to adapt or grow stronger. It has been established that all of the benefits of strength training can be obtained in as little as one two to five minute workout per week—but it doesn't take an Alan Greenspan to figure out that there is more money to be made from a client who is willing and has the depth of pockets to pay to have you train him for twenty hours a week, rather than five minutes a week. It must be pointed out that Tiger Woods was an exceptional golfer long before he started strength training and that whatever benefit he might be obtaining in the gym pales in comparison to the advantages he has developed through neural training (i.e., practice—hitting golf balls, developing his swing, playing the game of golf) and genetics. It bears repeating, nobody needs to work out twenty hours a week—nobody—and certainly not a golfer. This is not a prescription for building superior strength and improving one's game of golf; this is a prescription for bone-crippling osteoarthritis by the time Tiger hits his late forties or early fifties.

Q: I understand what you're saying about muscle and its relationship to moving our limbs as we hit golf balls. However, I also think that the "inner game" of golf (i.e., the mind set, focus, etc.) is important.

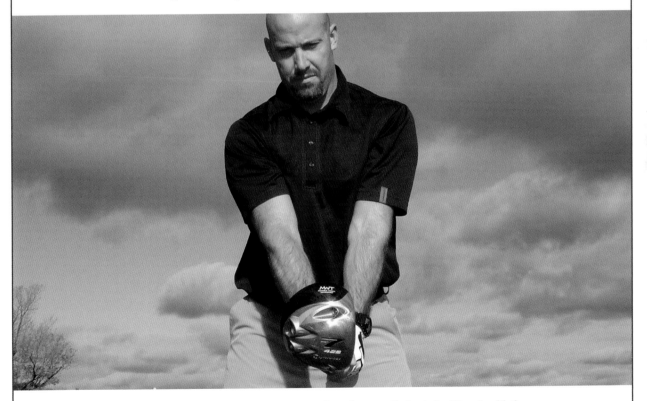

The mind and body are interconnected as a fact of nature. Trying to feel "one" with the universe is fine (if you're into that), but it's not necessary to improve your game of golf.

You don't seem to address this point. What are your thoughts on the mental aspects of golf?

A: The mind and body are interconnected. Indeed, the mind, per se, is enclosed in the brain, which is a physical organ, not unlike your pancreas, and therefore is very much a part of the body. You are not, therefore, a de-cerebrated body, nor a disembodied mind. I do not subscribe to any sort of "Zen" state of mind as being necessary for golfing success, as not only is there little to no evidence supporting such a contention, but there have been too many successful golfers who don't engage in any such mental gymnastics to shoot an exceptional round of golf (and even win Masters Championships).

Unquestionably, the most common arguments that you'll encounter are the "visualization" or cognitive "mind over matter" arguments. These are, in effect, mind over genetics arguments. You're instructed to ignore the fact that you're only five foot two and have brown eyes because, by God, if you really want to be six foot six and have eyes of blue then all you have to do is *believe that it's possible*—and it will happen! The proponents of such irrational gibberish have their own nomenclature, featuring terms such as "*mental imagery*" or "*visualization*"—and it's rampant throughout the golf world. Statements like "Believe and Achieve" adorn the back of many personally inscribed golf bags—but the truth is this is chicanery straight out of *The Flim-Flam Man*—and won't put another inch on your drive, no matter how "clear and distinct" your thoughts about your tee shot resulting in a hole-in-one may be. I mean, go ahead—envision driving your golf ball over the peak of Mt. Everest—give me a call when it reaches 29,028 feet above sea level.

If "believe and achieve" were true, then those deranged individuals who sincerely believe that they're Napoleon would be Napoleon—simply as a result of their believing it to be true. Likewise, if a golfer of international repute should tell you that he has added twenty yards to his drive—not because he has gotten stronger (after all, it is muscle strength that contributes to the velocity of the club head)—but because he saw in a Zen-like trance that his ball traveled sixty feet further, you should be equally suspect about his cognitive faculties. Nevertheless, such claims are made on an almost daily basis regarding the mystical import of the "mind" in golf. Sure, the mind is important. Without it you couldn't even tie your shoes let alone engage in swinging a golf club, but the mind is not nearly as omnipotent as some "authorities" would have you believe.

The mind is important in keeping you motivated to get into the gym and train intensely enough to stimulate your muscles to grow stronger—which, as I have discussed in previous chapters—is not an easy task (particularly as you grow stronger and the energy drain you face each workout grows greater). In fact, it's downright uncomfortable. So much so, in fact, that anyone who feels the inclination to engage in "visualization" or cognitive gymnastics really isn't training—they're simply going through the motions and relaxing, because relaxation or "sleep" is the time we are best able to engage in such flights of fancy (we just refer to them as dreams).

Q: You're correct that training to the max is difficult. How do you stay motivated to give 100 percent of your energy to the task of working out year after year?

A: The ethos of Max Contraction Training is: be willing to give 100 percent of what you have to a given task. It is the cornerstone of my personal philosophy, and those of others who have likewise embraced this method of training. Stated another way, the concept is that if you are going to attempt anything, then give it everything you've got—or don't bother. Nobody in life benefits from a half-assed effort: not in work (employer and employee), not in love (where neither party has a maximum emotional investment), and certainly not in exercise (which must be intense enough to stimulate an adaptive response). When we are able to transcend, if only by a degree, our previous levels of effort and energy output, we invariably make quantum leaps in progress. These Max efforts help us break through to higher functional levels, and, as a result, they are powerful learning experiences that teach us much about our physical and intellectual potential.

According to psychologist William James, "Compared with what we ought to be, we are only half awake. Our fires are damped, our drafts are checked. We are making use of only a small part of our possible mental and physical resources." All of us, in other words, operate well within our existing limits, failing—as William James might say—to make full use of the power we know we possess. Our day-to-day existence is typified by this reluctance to engage in an all-out physical effort; it's something that is ordinarily avoided when possible. As mentioned earlier, we are a species that has survived owing to a cultivated ability to conserve—rather than expend—energy. Consequently, other than in athletic competition, such effort is produced typically in emergency situations only. Only a person fired by a strong, almost overwhelming sense of purpose and meaning will be able to train his muscles to the point where he has tapped all of their energy.

So, the question becomes: how strong is the value you place on getting stronger? On getting leaner? On becoming a better golfer? If it's not that strong, then the reality is that you will not be able to moti-

Seeing constant improvement in your strength (and its positive effects on your golf game) will often serve as sufficient motivational fuel to ensure that you continue to give your all to each workout you perform.

vate yourself sufficiently to generate the kind of effort level necessary to move you closer to your goal. If you value these things highly enough, then motivation and effort (and results) will never be a problem. Former Mr. Universe winner Mike Mentzer, who taught me much about productive exercise, once pointed out that

> Nature does not allow living creatures to be inactive. In all levels of biology, inactivity spells death. Life is growing: When not moving forward, it falls backward. We survive, then, only as long as we advance. Humankind evolved through continuous struggle and effort. Since men and women are distinguished from other creatures because they have a mind, they will get the best out of themselves when they employ their rational ability to focus on the future, that is, attaining their goals. The individual who wants to evolve physically and mentally must be willing to exert continuous effort.

> Since life by its nature involves struggle, we are also faced with the constant possibility of defeat. Hence, humankind derives intense pleasure from successful effort, as it confirms the possibility of success in life. An individual's self-esteem stems from a sense of control over reality. Whenever we carry out a conscious effort, such as when we struggle against an opposing force like doing a 400-pound bench press, we feel a specific power rising in us, a sense of "will." The abundant self-esteem associated with champion bodybuilders stems precisely from their having achieved goals by generating the proper effort. They took the time and expended the necessary energy to develop their self-respect. They sufficiently value life and happiness to exert complete effort. As a result they rightfully feel pride.

> Individuals who avoid effort may end up with problems stemming from the meaning and value they attach to life. The chronic avoidance of effort eventually will cause the person's inner resources to atrophy. This sense of impotence in life can make such individuals feel helpless in the face of even minor adversities.

Q: I find the thought of working out once a week very appealing—and quite revolutionary. Are there any other studies that have been performed on the effects of once a week training that I could read up on?

A: Yes. Two come to mind right away:

1. Graves, J. E., et al. "Effect of reduced training frequency on muscular strength." *International Journal of Sports Medicine* 9 (5):316–319, 1988.
2. DeRenne, C. "Effects of training frequency on strength maintenance in pubescent baseball players." *Journal of Strength and Conditioning Research* 10 (1):8–14, 1996.

In both of these studies they essentially they took groups of subjects that were training three days a week and two days a week, and looked at their rate of progress. And then the group that was training three times a week was cut back to training two times a week, and the group

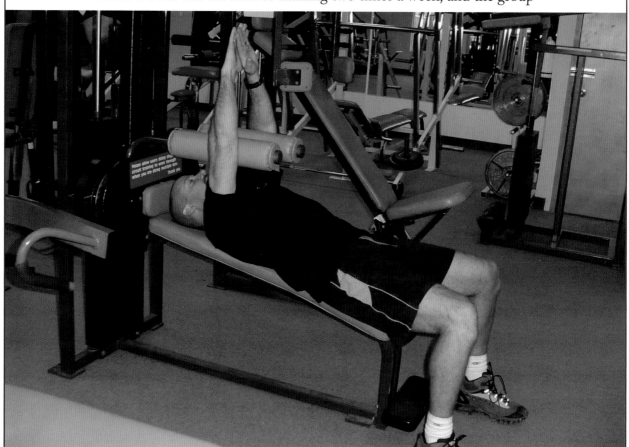

There is no valid scientific basis for engaging in strength training more often than once a week.

that was training two times a week, was cut back to one time a week. And in doing so the experimenters noted that the subjects' rate of progress improved. And there have been other similar studies; this has been duplicated in other studies in different age subjects wherein the experimenters take them and decrease their training frequency and find that they actually do better—particularly the elderly. But even in younger subjects this is borne out. Regarding seniors, the Academic Health Care Center of the New York College of Osteopathic Medicine and the Department of Physical Therapy, New York Institute of Technology, School of Health Professions, Behavioral and Life Sciences, published a study comparing the results of seniors training once a week and seniors training twice a week, and found, in their words, "no difference in strength changes between training once a week versus twice a week after 9 weeks. . . . One set of exercises performed once weekly to muscle fatigue improved strength as well as twice a week in the older adult." There are more data coming in each year to support the fact that training more than once a week represents nothing more than more time needlessly spent in a gym.

For instance, the May 1993 edition of the *Journal of Physiology* contained a report about a group of men and women aged twenty-two to thirty-two who took part in an exercise experiment in which they trained only their biceps muscles in a negative-only fashion to a point of muscular failure. Negative or eccentric contractions (which consist of lowering—rather than raising or lifting—the resistance) are considered by some exercise physiologists to be more intense than positive or concentric contractions because of the fact that more weight can be employed and, thus, the intensity of the exercise can be increased. All of the test subjects were found to be most sore two days after exercising (a common occurrence by the way) but the soreness in their biceps was gone by the ninth day. However, what was even more telling was not the highly subjective report of "soreness" in the muscles, but the far more tangible report of the impact of the workout on their strength levels. The day after the exercise the subjects exhibited what the experimenters termed "a dramatic 35% loss of strength. . . . even on the tenth post-exercise day the muscles had recovered only to about 70% of their control strength."

The experimenters, John N. Howell, Gary Chleboun, and Robert Conaster (from the Somatic Dysfunction Research Laboratory of the College of Osteopathic Medicine and the Department of Biological Sciences at Ohio University, Athens) concluded in their summary that "muscle strength declined by almost 40% after the exercise and recovery was only slight 10 days later; the half-time of recovery appeared to be as long as 5–6 weeks."

Given that a muscle must recover before it overcompensates or adapts, the positive change a trainee is seeking from exercise will only arrive after full recovery has taken place, meaning that many weeks "off" from training will be required before the benefit (the adaptation from the workout) can be produced. And lest you think that overtraining is of concern only to those who engage in heavy strength training, additional research conducted on marathon runners (who engage in highly repetitive, lower intensity activity) by Michael Sherman at Ball State University in Indiana also indicated that the recovery period required after even low intensity (high volume) training can extend to a period running into months. In the January 1985 issue of *American Health* magazine, Stephen Kiesling reported that "Sherman found that even after a full week of rest, marathon runners had not regained pre-race strength and power. Returning to [even] moderate running after the marathon delayed recovery. And some races may take months to recover from."

It is also worth pointing out that the iconic runner Roger Bannister revealed in the December 1996 edition of *Runner's World* magazine that he in fact *rested for five full days* prior to his breaking the four-minute mile barrier. Bannister believed that *not* running during those days prior to the race allowed him to take his mind off the competition, but from the research cited above, his days of rest actually allowed his body additional time to recover from his running sessions and his recuperative subsystems to replenish and grow stronger, thus allowing him to run the first-ever sub-four-minute mile.

In seriously considering the data cited above, we are forced to conclude that the recovery process can take not one to two weeks, but quite possibly up to ten to twelve weeks! That is to say, up to three months off might be required in order to simply recover from an intense workout.

The conclusion to draw from the data cited above (as well as what I indicated in previous chapters) is simply that training—of almost any variety—creates far greater demands on the body's recuperative subsystems than most people (including many strength coaches and personal trainers) realize. Muscular adaptation is a biological process, and therefore it is not mediated by traditional societal considerations such as the Gregorian calendar with its seven-day week. Adding additional muscle to your body and improving your fitness level is not an easy process (if it were, there would be a lot more fit and muscular—and a lot less overweight—people running about the fairways), with the result that you cannot force your body to become fitter and stronger by subjecting it to marathon-style low intensity training (mild exertion) sessions. As your body can already handle this level of intensity, there is no reason for it to alter its present level of fitness and strength. Your objective in training—whether it is to lose fat, tone up, strengthen your muscles, protect your joints and connective tissues to enhance mobility or athletic performance, or simply to look better—will never be realized by training geared to seeing how much exercise you can tolerate, nor how many different exercise sessions you can squeeze into a seven-day period.

Like medicine, exercise must be applied in the correct dose and the correct frequency in order to produce the optimal response from your body. Any more than the precise amount required will result in your body "overdosing" on the stimulus, which can take many months to recover from. When it comes to exercise, "more" isn't better. Any amount more than the least amount required to realize your objectives is overtraining, by definition.

In conclusion, then, it would appear that the best exercise one could perform—no matter what one's personal choice in exercise—is the exercise of restraint.

Q: If I grow stronger, can't I perform more exercise? I'm not clear on how a more advanced trainee can benefit from performing less exercise. Please explain.

A: Bear in mind that as an individual grows bigger and stronger, his or her energy output increases proportionally, as the heavier the resistance that the muscles are made to contract against, the greater the energy output that is required to perform these heavier contractions, and the longer it takes these energy reserves of the human body to replenish themselves. Golfers who ignore or otherwise fail to make their peace with this biological law will soon see their strength training progress grind to a halt. The only way such plateaus or sticking points can be obviated is if the golfer continues to make the requisite adjustment (in the form of adding additional "rest" or "recovery" days into his training schedule) to compensate for the increasing demands of the training stress to which he is subjecting his system.

The reason being that each time an individual becomes stronger, he has increased the intensity of his workout, and each time the intensity of his workout is increased, the longer it takes the body to put back what was used up (and more time must be allotted for overcompensation—the

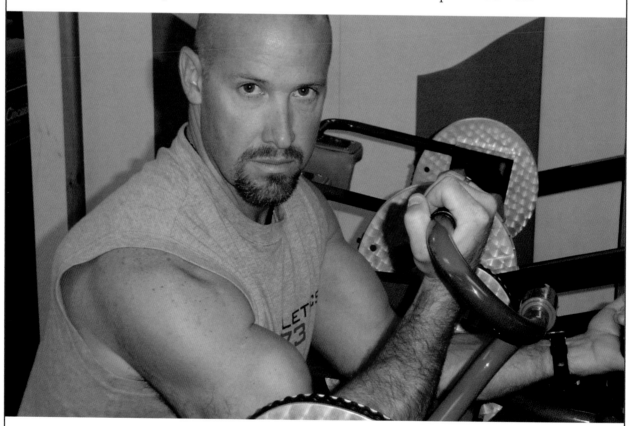

As you grow stronger, you simply use up more energy more quickly. You don't, however, replenish your energy reserves quicker. Consequently, as you grow stronger you need to train less frequently.

strength gain—to take place). Additionally, each time one increases the intensity of one's workout, a corresponding adjustment must be made to the volume of his effort during the workout. For the same reason that an all-out sprint is more intense than a walk, it cannot be continued for as long a period of time (i.e., you can walk for miles but only sprint for a handful of yards). The same is true with strength training exercise; i.e., the more intense the workout, the shorter its duration has to be.

When one is a beginner, the stress one is capable of generating and thus subjecting one's muscles to is minimal, with the result that one has the luxury of being able to endure repeated exposure to such a low intensity training stress (e.g., training with many sets, many days per week, and many routines, if one so desires) and will make progress—perhaps not as significant progress as he would make if he trained more intensely, but then again, a twelve-inch arm contracting maximally does not place the same demands on the body's energy systems as does a fifteen-inch arm contracting maximally. A beginner's muscles are literally too "weak" to generate the intensity required to thoroughly tax the body's energy systems so as to prevent recovery from occurring between training sessions. However, as the beginner becomes stronger, his energy output and ability to raise the stress he can subject his muscles to increases (in some instances quite dramatically), with the result that he quickly finds that he can no longer recover and grow stronger in twenty-four hours, forty-eight hours, seventy-two hours—or even longer. It is at this juncture in his training career that the trainee should begin to insert additional "off" or "rest" days into his routine and to reduce the duration of his exposure to the training stress.

This last point is one of the most crucially important elements of exercise science, and has been completely overlooked by almost everyone. With very few exceptions, almost every personal trainer has his clients stay on the same volume and frequency protocol virtually forever. Once the fundamental principles are understood, however, the issue of progressively decreasing the volume and, especially, the frequency of one's training becomes the most pressing issue. If the trainee bears this in mind, he will never reach a sticking point, there will be no need to engage in such protocols as "periodization" (wherein you train efficiently, i.e., intensely, for certain periods of time and then train inefficiently, i.e., with less intensity, for other periods), and he will actualize his full strength and muscular potential in a relatively short time.

Q: Do you think that it's a good idea to do a little bit more abdominal work—to really strengthen the "core" muscles better? I believe that they contribute to trunk rotation, which would be helpful in golf.

A: The so-called "core" muscles are the abdominals. And as the function of the abdominal muscles is to draw the trunk toward the thighs, this action is perfectly covered with the Max Crunch exercise using Max Straps. Once you've drained the energy out of the abdominal muscles in this fashion, there is nothing else, in terms of exercise, that is required to strengthen them. It must be remembered that the abdominals are skeletal muscles—just like the biceps and calves—and, therefore, their training requirement is no different from these other muscle groups. The abdominals don't require volume training but rather high-intensity training, which, as we know, must be intense, brief, and infrequent. Training your muscles in this manner will result in superb abdominal strength. Rely on practicing your swing to perfect your technique. Incidentally, trunk rotation is actually a function of the oblique muscles and the hips, with the abdominals contributing very little to the action.

Q: I recently bought your audio lectures and read your book—terrific information. However, I did not see anywhere what you recommend for preparation, such as warm ups, stretching out, etc. It would seem unreasonable to come into the gym and start lifting a max weight without some sort of warm up?

A: Warm ups are very important, but also a very individual-oriented phenomenon, depending on such things as the individual's age, existing physical condition, prior training history, and injury history. For these reasons, it is difficult for anyone to prescribe such a program without dealing with each trainee on an individual basis. Typically warm ups are required for full-range or conventional training, as you are moving a weight throughout a full range of motion and, as the weights get heavier (for your working set), the potential shear forces on joints and connective tissue increases. As Max Contraction is motionless exercise, and the exercise that is performed is executed in your strongest range of motion (i.e., where your leverage is optimal and your muscles, joints, and connective tissues are strongest and, thus, best able to accommodate it),

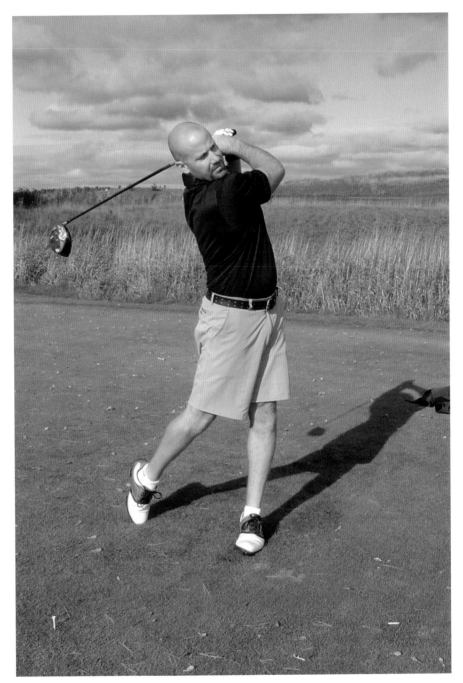

It is not necessary to perform an obsessive amount of "core" or abdominal exercise in order to enhance trunk rotation during your swing.

a warm-up is not always required. Having said this, if you are training with conventional Max Contraction you may wish to perform three or four progressive "holds" wherein you simply increase the resistance and hold it for one or two seconds. This should only be required for the first two or three exercises in a given workout; thereafter, your body temperature should be elevated sufficiently to have provided an adequate "warm up" for the remaining body parts.

Q: I can understand that one set of an exercise is sufficient to stimulate muscle growth (all of the scientific studies you presented in your first book, *Max Contraction Training*, made this obvious), but I'm still having trouble wrapping my mind around the concept that one

The need to warm-up prior to exercise is not a bad idea if you have an history of injury.

repetition is enough to stimulate muscle growth. Is there any scientific basis for this?

A: Yes. Apart from my own research, I also cited the ten-year study performed by Dr. Muller from Germany. Not only did he establish that only one set was required to stimulate size and strength increases, but also that a single contraction (or "rep," if you will) was sufficient for this same purpose. More recently, the research of a physiologist named Berger was brought to my attention. Over fifty years ago, Berger, tested various training protocols to determine if any were inherently superior in stimulating size and strength increases. Berger experimented with untrained male students whom he taught at college. After a three-week break-in period in which the subjects were taught the mechanics of

One maximal contraction is all that is required to induce optimal muscle size and strength stimulation.

the squat exercise and to allow for neuromuscular or motor learning, several classes (rather than individual students) were randomly assigned to seven experimental groups, each training with a variant of the One-Rep Max protocol. Each group performed *one repetition* of the squat across the six weeks of this phase of the study. The first group did 66 percent of their 1-RM twice per week; group two did 80 percent of their 1-RM twice per week; group three used 90 percent of their 1-RM twice per week; group four used 100 percent of their 1-RM twice per week; group five used 66 percent of their 1-RM three times per week; group six only trained once per week and did a 1-RM, while group seven was a control group and did not train at all. Berger's conclusion was that "training once weekly with a 1-RM was considered as effective for increasing strength as either training twice weekly with various proportions of the 1-RM, and once weekly with the 1-RM, or three times weekly with the 1-RM."

If one maximum repetition stimulated the same size and strength increase as did protocols employing more than one repetition, it reveals the absolute non-necessity of engaging in these other protocols.

Q: In your book and Max Contraction Training DVD you illustrate the use of a training tool called "Max Straps." I like to do Max Contraction Training, but I also like full range training. Can Max Straps be utilized in conventional bodybuilding workouts?

A: Certainly. While Max Straps were created specifically for Max Contraction trainees, they can be used for all types of bodybuilding training and have been employed to great effect with hundreds of clients. And while I do illustrate how to use Max Straps in my book and training DVD, you will also find that I have listed alternative exercises to the ones where Max Straps are indicated for those who do not have access to these straps, so there are alternatives. Nautilus machines (the older ones preferably) are very effective in isolating the lats, such as their Pullover, Super Pullover, and Behind Neck machines—however, you will find that these pieces of "isolation" equipment are far more expensive than the economical version I am promoting (i.e., several thousand dollars versus $69). Remember, the more you can make an exercise direct, i.e., the more ancillary muscle groups you can take out of the exercise, the better and more thorough the stimulation of the particular muscle

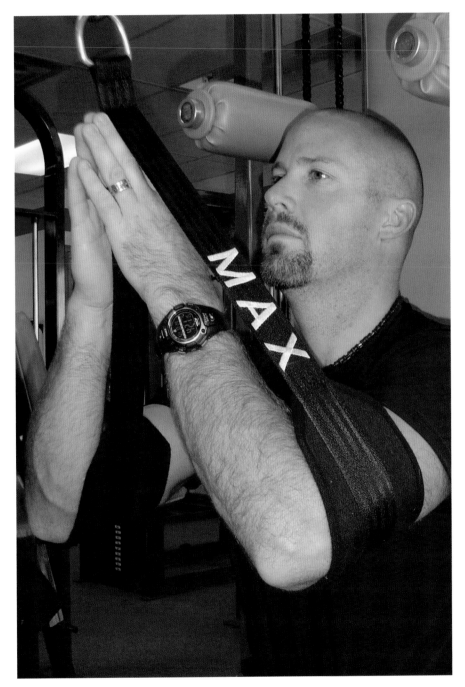

Max Straps provide direct resistance to the muscle being worked (in this instance, the latissimus dorsi muscles of the upper back), resulting in a greater degree of growth stimulation.

group you are attempting to train. Max Straps do this very efficiently and so are featured in the book and training DVD for that reason. For those bodybuilders who wish to learn more about Max Straps, please visit Max Contraction online at www.maxcontraction.com.

Q: It is widely known that strength increases as the result of isometrics are joint angle specific, in that the strength increases only occur at the angle the contraction was held at. In your book you suggest taking a joint to the end of its range of motion so that the muscle is in a fully contracted position, and then applying isometric tension at this point. My question is, will this method allow uniform strength to be gained throughout the full range of motion, or will it still be restricted to the joint angle, in your case at the end of the range of motion?

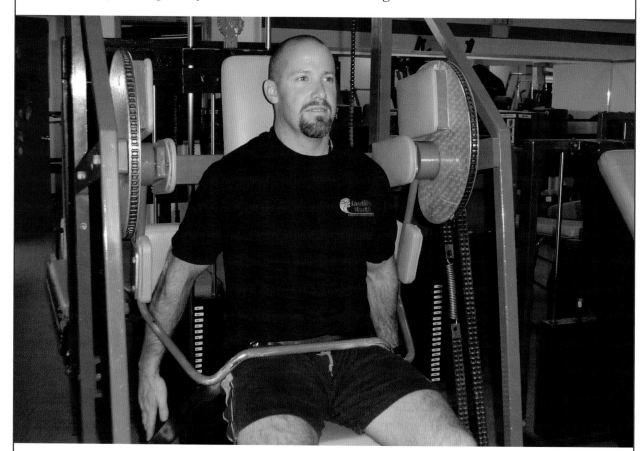

Full contraction—not full range—is the most important factor for strengthening muscles.

A: I, too, have heard about the alleged "non-transference" of strength increases in one's strongest range to one's full range. I believe Arthur Jones even conducted some testing in the 1980s on this, but that he found that only *some* (whom he dubbed to be type "S" or "specific") did not record a transference of strength from one position of flexion to full range. Others, whom he classified as type "G" (for "general") did record a positive transfer to full range strength after training exclusively—and statically—in one position. However, my answer to your question would be in two parts.

First, the primary factor in muscle fiber recruitment and, thus, muscle fiber stimulation, is the intensity of the contraction of a given muscle. That is, how heavy the load is that your muscles are made to contract against, with the heavier load requiring more fibers to accomplish the task of contraction. It used to be believed that if you trained a muscle "through a full range of motion" you would be "training the full muscle," whereas if you "trained a muscle in one position, you would only be developing one part of the muscle," when actually the reverse is true; i.e., if you train through a full range of motion, then you will only develop part of the muscle, predominantly slow twitch and intermediate twitch fibers, as those are the only fibers that can be recruited owing to the fact that a full range of motion restricts you to using a lighter weight than what you are actually capable of maximally contracting against. As muscle fibers are recruited solely by the amount of force they must produce (i.e., the amount of weight they are made to contract against), and as you are capable of contracting against more weight in the fully contracted position than you are restricted to using in your weakest range of motion, you will recruit and therefore stimulate all fibers (i.e., the full muscle) with a Max Contraction set.

Muscles contract by shortening or reducing their length, therefore the one position where all of the fibers are contracted would be (by definition) the "fully contracted position" (what I term the position of "Max Contraction"). In other words, the two factors responsible for maximal stimulation of a given muscle both involve "maximums"; i.e., that the muscle be in a maximally contracted position and that the load imposed on the muscle while in this position be the maximum that the muscle is capable of contracting against. This said, what fibers would not be recruited from this protocol? If all the fibers are recruited as a result of the two requisites indicated, then that would include the fibers involved during the first sixteenth of contraction, the first quarter of contraction, the first third of contraction, the first half of contraction, the third quarter of contraction, and so on—as all of these same fibers are involved in the shortening or "contracting" process. As a result, all fibers that can be stimulated to grow stronger will have been stimulated to grow stronger from a "zero" range of motion—providing this zero range of motion takes place in the muscle's fully contracted position. Jones, to my knowledge, tested his subjects at different points in the range of motion and, as the fully contracted position is the only position where all of the fibers are brought together and where, indeed, the contraction can only be said to be truly "maximal," it is not surprising that a weak range contraction would produce results only proportionate to the amount of fibers recruited and stimulated in that range. Any other point but that of maximum contraction is by definition a sub-maximum contraction, and hence less productive. I would also mention that Peter Sisco conducted an informal study with motionless (static) exercise and determined that there was a 35 percent transference of strength to full range or dynamic strength. It might be argued that 35 percent proves that a full transference of strength did not take place, but when you consider that none of these trainees on the study had gained any strength using full-range of motion exercise for several months prior to performing the static holds, a 35 percent increase in their full-range positive strength is considerable. Second, I don't believe an increase in full range of motion strength to be the benchmark that many others believe it to be. If you increase your strength in a given position by 80 percent, and you gain seventeen pounds of muscle in the process, you would obviously be accomplishing your objective of building a bigger, stronger body. The fact that this can be accomplished in so little time (seconds a week versus the hours a week required by conventional approaches) means that this is a more efficient means of achieving your objective. And unless you absolutely require the ability to bench press throughout a full range of motion many hundreds of pounds on a progressive basis, what would be the point of devoting hours and years to the cultivation of this talent? You don't need to do this to become bigger and stronger; indeed, it is actually an impediment to becoming bigger and stronger as a full range of motion actually reduces the amount of resistance your muscles are capable of contracting maximally against, thus providing sub-maximal overload (and results) to your muscles. Training throughout a full range of motion does NOT (again, contrary to the popular view) enhance flexibility (which has a strong genetically mediated limit to begin with; i.e., a muscle cannot "increase" its flexibility without either tearing something or losing its tonus) more thoroughly than performing a Max Contraction (as the stronger the muscle—the whole muscle—the more secure the joint and mechano-receptor sites responsible for tonus/tension and relaxation or stretch). Indeed, there is ample evidence that training with moderately heavy weights throughout a full range of motion will actually increase your chance of injury owing the sheer forces that impinge on joints and connective tissue when bones and ligaments are required to move through arcs and positions of disadvantaged leverage.

If your objective in training is to have a stronger full range of motion (that is, to be able to lift heavier weights through a full range of motion), the best approach would be to train specifically for this skill—by performing only full range movements. This will, however, severely compromise your ability to build maximum size and strength in your muscles as, again, your muscles are capable of contracting against much heavier weights than a full range of motion allows you to employ. And the heavier the weights, the more intense the contraction, and the more intense the contraction (when combined with proper rest periods), the greater the muscle growth production.

Q: Muscle fibers don't usually run the length of a muscle. So if you only build the fibers in an isolated part of the muscle, you don't build all the fibers above and below it. And that just has to limit your muscle growth, right? This is one law of exercise physiology you can't sidestep.

A: I won't sidestep it, but meet it head on. This is a specious argument because motor units distribute their fibers homogeneously throughout the length of a muscle. So when you recruit motor units, you do so homogeneously throughout the whole distribution of the muscle. The nerves that enter a given muscle divide out into threads that resemble branches on a tree. Each branch ends at the muscle cell and carries the electrochemical current that causes each muscle cell to contract. When

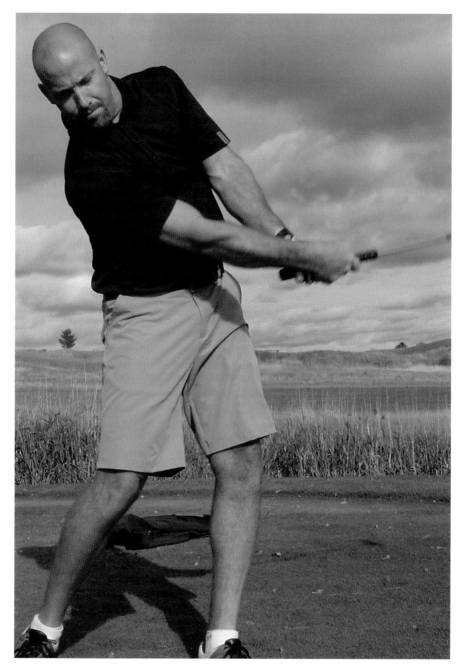

The notion that training with Max Contraction will only develop the muscle and strength and size in the range in which the contraction is performed is specious because motor units (groups of muscle fibers) distribute their fibers homogenously throughout the entire length of a muscle.

this current is released, all of the cells serviced by the branch (a single neuron) contract simultaneously (the all-or-none law of muscle fiber contraction), not some to the exclusion of others. It's simply not possible to isolate one portion, border, or ridge of a muscle. But don't take my word for it. Consider this excerpt from Dr. Fred Hatfield's book on *Bodybuilding: A Scientific Approach*:

> The cells associated with each motor unit are spread all through the gross muscle; all portions of the gross muscle are affected similarly by a given exercise and therefore develop similarly. This is called the principle of noncontiguous innervation. Using many variations of an exercise for one muscle in no way ensures more growth or different growth patterning than does performing the basic exercise. . . . The shape of that muscle will not be affected by variations in the angle or position of stress application. Does this mean that all a bodybuilder has to do is perform the basic movement and rid himself or herself of the array of supplemental exercises for a given muscle? I suspect it does.

Q: Were the subjects in the Nautilus North study regaining previously held muscle mass?

A: No. The subjects who took part in the Nautilus North study had been training steadily for a period of at least six months with high intensity protocols and had been training only once a week in this fashion prior to the study. None of them were regaining previously held muscle mass but were hopeful to build new muscle mass. The subjects in the Nautilus North study were not grossly underweight or overweight, nor were they under-conditioned, being instead young to middle-aged men, several of whom were fresh out of college where they ran track and participated in activities such as football, hockey, and martial arts. They were not previously over-trained and then able to take advantage of the two week testing period for recovery, and they were not made to drink lots of water before testing or to eat any particular diet beyond what they normally consumed on a daily basis and had been consuming for the previous several months prior to the study being conducted. These were simply fit, and, in some cases, already very strong individuals who had an

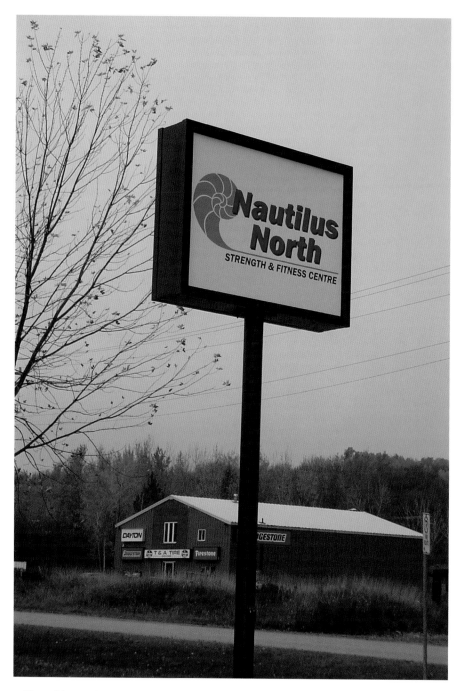

The subjects who took part in the Nautilus North Study were building new muscle mass, rather than regaining previously held muscle mass.

interest in seeing what effect a high intensity workout had on the body and what if any gains could be produced from a solitary workout. As the subjects would not be regaining previously held muscle mass and were already fairly well developed regarding their individual genetic potential for mass and strength, any gains were noteworthy and of significance to those interested in building new muscle from exercise.

Q: I'm still not clear on the whole issue of recovery ability. Are you saying that everyone now only needs to train once a week?

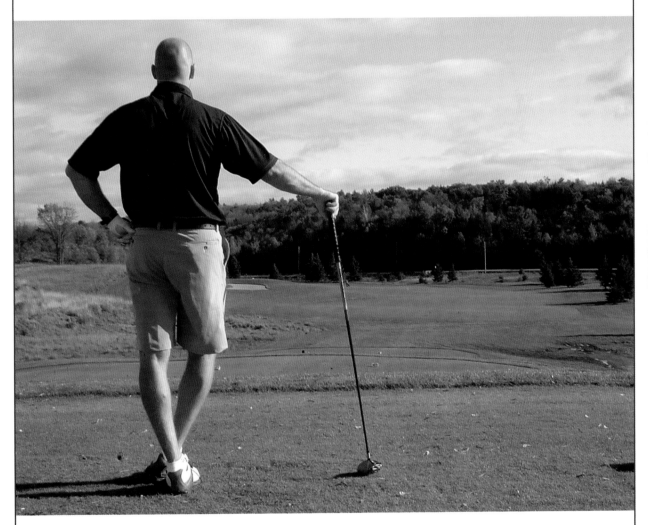

Golf as often as you wish—strength train as little as is required.

A: What I'm saying is that as you get stronger, you will need to train less frequently. You might think of it this way: When a beginner works out it takes "X" units of time to recover from the workout, an intermediate trainee with his greater energy expenditure will require "Y" units of time, and the advanced trainee requires "Z" units of time. We should get out of the rut of thinking in terms of seven-day periods—particularly in matters pertaining to human biology. The body simply requires the amount of time that it requires (which will vary beyond the confines of the seven-day week) to recover from the stress of exercise. The measurement/recovery method is out of date with the new model of fitness. Perhaps a more accurate measurement would be to start at "A" units of time, and then every time that an individual grows stronger, assume that it will simply take more units of time for full recovery—and then over-compensation or adaptation—to take place. Training within the confines of a week works well for beginners but not because it is a two-day or seven-day interval, but because the beginner's recovery happens to fall into this realm of time—the advanced trainee's does not. In 1971 Arthur Jones made the statement in his *Nautilus Bulletin #2* that

> When anything is in limited supply, then it is simply common-sense practice to make the best-possible utilization of the quantity that is available—and when you are not sure just how much is available, it is equally good practice to use as little as necessary; in the field of exercise, the implication is clear—use your limited recovery ability as wisely as possible, and as little as possible in line with the actual requirements for producing the results you are after.

This is absolutely true. And as your limited supply of recovery ability does not get bigger, but the demands you are placing on your muscles and energy systems do, it only stands to reason to disturb your limited reserve of recovery resources as sparingly as possible by training only as much as is required—not as many times as you can fit into an arbitrary time period such as seven days.

Q: One of the strength coaches at my university has the football players training with plyometrics, where they jump with weights and perform their repetitions as quickly as possible to become explosive. What are your thoughts on this method of training for golfers? Will it make me more explosive off the tee?

A: The facts of the matter regarding impact forces and the nature of muscle fiber recruitment obviously fly in the face of what some of the bodybuilding and strength coaches have been preaching regarding plyometrics and other such "explosive" movements for developing

Make your body stronger through proper strength training—and then take that stronger you onto the course and play golf. Trying to train "explosively" will only lead to excess forces being placed on your joints and connective tissues, and could well result in your missing golfing opportunities because of needlessly incurred injuries.

strength and muscle size. Their theories, that the "fast-twitch" muscle fibers can only be activated by performing various exercises as fast as you possibly can, have been shown to be fallacious in light of what science has revealed regarding the principles of motor control and muscle fiber recruitment. First off, if you train utilizing a very high rate of speed and ballistic movements, you will be forced to use light weights as, the heavier the resistance, the slower you can move it. If you use a light weight, the brain immediately picks up on the FORCE required to move that weight and, obviously, with a light weight, the FORCE required to move the resistance at a high speed would prove sufficient to engage the "S" (slow twitch) and maybe the "FO" (fast oxidative or intermediate twitch) fibers. The "FG" (fast-twitch glyco-lytic) fibers—the ones most important to high speed movement and the one's contributing the most to increases in size and strength—are never activated in such a system because the resistance you will have restricted yourself to using will not be sufficient to warrant the brain sending the signal to recruit the "FGs" that would otherwise engage the full complement of muscle fibers. Not only does ballistic or ply-ometric training not stimulate the muscle fibers its theory purports it does, but it only involves half of the muscle fibers available to be stimulated in any given set. Obviously if you're only stimulating half the fibers you could be, your training system is only half as efficient as it could be, and certainly only half as efficient as Max Contraction Training, which engages all of the available muscle fibers (right down to the FG fibers). Any training system that is predicated on heaving weights up and down ballistically will not even come close to bringing the target muscle group into a position of full-muscular contraction for any meaningful length of time and certainly will not engage anywhere near the full complement of available muscle fibers. As if that wasn't enough, such training is highly traumatic to your joints and connective tissues. A barbell weighing 100 pounds, for example, if curled slowly in the conventional fashion will provide 100 pounds of resistance both concentrically and eccentrically (up and down). Holding 100 pounds in a position of full muscular contraction will do likewise. However, jerking and heaving that same 100-pound barbell up and down will magnify the trauma force on the joints to well over 1,000 pounds—and the impact to the joints which must suddenly stretch and then ballistically extend muscles, tendons, ligaments, and muscle fascia, can quickly add up to injury. Again, high-speed training is dangerous and far less productive than Max Contraction Training.

Q: I've heard that isometric type exercises can cause an increase in blood pressure. If so, doesn't this make Max Contraction and other "static" type exercise protocols more dangerous than regular training?

A: The truth is that your blood pressure goes up during any vigorous exercise of any sort, including cycling, cross-country skiing, running, calisthenics, and weight training. In the textbook entitled *Exercise Physiology* by Professors William D. McArdle, Frank I. Katch, and Victor L. Katch, they tested isometric or "motionless" exercise against two modes of isotonic exercise. The study was conducted at the University of Massachusetts and the blood pressure of normotensive subjects was measured directly with a pressure transducer connected to a catheter that was inserted into the femoral artery. They then tested the blood pressure response of the subject performing four sets of isometric bench

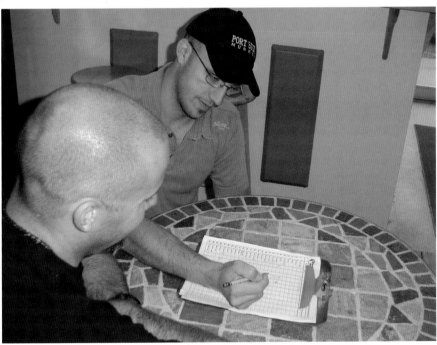

Max Contraction training is actually less risky than other forms of exercise.

presses at 25, 50, 75, and 100 percent of maximal voluntary contraction in the same arm and body position as the two other protocols, which were free weight bench presses performed at 25 and 50 percent of the maximum voluntary contraction and a hydraulic resistance bench press performed "all-out" for twenty seconds' duration at two settings: slow (for eleven reps) and fast (for sixteen reps) carried through a full range of motion.

According to the textbook, all three forms of exercise produced dramatic elevations in blood pressure—even with relatively light exercise that required only 25 percent of the maximal effort. In looking over the data myself, I note that the peak systolic and peak diastolic conditions were actually somewhat higher with the full range exercises than with the isometric exercise (at 100 percent contraction isometrically, the peak systolic was 225 and the peak diastolic was 156, compared with 232 and 154 for the free weight full-range bench press and 245 and 160 for the hydraulic full range bench press). This makes sense, of course, because it doesn't take a maximal effort to cause an increase in blood pressure. In fact, your blood pressure is probably rising right now from the sodium in the soft drink you're drinking. Many common everyday tasks like carrying a briefcase and maintaining your posture are largely static or isometric and not considered "dangerous."

It's interesting to note that the increase in blood pressure from full-range weight training was one of the reasons that Arthur Jones designed his Nautilus equipment the way he did and why he also stressed that you should not grip the handles of the machines too tightly when training. This is not to trivialize the concern—it is important that anyone beginning a vigorous weight training program get his or her physician's okay beforehand. But it's also a fact that any increase in blood pressure from weight training exercise such as Max Contraction returns to normal quite quickly after you complete your workout provided that your cardiovascular system is functioning normally. James Wright, Ph.D., in an article on motionless exercise—the same one that premiered my training system to North American audiences back in 1992—wrote that isometrics or "static" exercise did not cause blood pressure increases that were any greater than conventional forms of weight training, writing:

. . . there is no evidence that the transient elevations that occur during [isometric] exercise persist or influence the development of hypertension or cardiovascular risk. . . . the blood pressure changes are no more—and no different—than those that occur during any kind of heavy lifting. That's one reason some physicians in years past weren't too keen on weightlifting and bodybuilding. But who can say that transient elevations in blood pressure—which only require the heart, which is a muscle, to pump harder for a brief period—is bad for you?

The idea that you can remove fat from one area of the body, such as the waist, by exercising it is a myth.

This said, individuals with a precondition to heart disease would obviously be at risk by engaging in any activity that elevates blood pressure—from swimming to weight training. And if you are one of these people, then Max Contraction Training would not be a wise thing to do—but it's no more dangerous and causes no greater increase in blood pressure than any other bodybuilding exercise. In fact, according to the study I just cited, it causes less of a blood pressure increase than conventional training.

Q: I would like to lose fat from the area around my chest and entire waist area without losing size anywhere else. Can I spot reduce these areas with Max Contraction?

A: Sorry to disillusion you, but "spot reduction" isn't physiologically possible; it is a bogus concept perpetrated by business interests selling "spot reduction" devices and supplements. When you go on a diet, fat will be mobilized from all of your body's multiple fat cells, not from isolated areas, such as those in the areas you might be exercising. Once fat has been broken down and mobilized it is transported by the blood to all the individual active cells in the body and burned for energy. You would be better advised to go on a general reducing diet in conjunction with Max Contraction Training, working all of your muscle groups in a single workout performed once to three times weekly. This will lower your overall percentage of body fat and build muscle at the same time, thereby causing a reduction in the areas you desire, while maintaining muscle size in all body parts.

Q: I like the idea of growing bigger and stronger muscles, but I've been told that should I ever stop training, all my muscles will turn to fat. What do you say to that?

A: I say that it's a supposition contrary to fact. Muscle and fat are two totally different types of tissue and one won't magically transform into the other any more than a peach will transform into a watermelon. Viewed under a microscope muscle is seen as long fibrous strands, known as myofibrils, while fat is comprised of little spherical globules. A chemical analysis of muscle and fat reveal the former to be made up of over 70 percent water, 6 percent lipids and about 22 percent protein. Fat, on the other hand is only 15 to 20 percent water, 70 percent lipids and approximately 15 percent protein. It's been a long standing false-hood that muscle turns to fat later in life, most likely arising from the

Muscle can't turn to fat anymore than a peach can turn into a watermelon; they are two different tissues.

fact that often times uneducated or just non-caring athletes would often continue eating the same quantity of food after they'd stopped competing as they did when they were competing. I knew many hockey players in Canada who were very lean when they were practicing several times a week and playing high-level hockey twice a week on top of this. Such a regimen required them to consume thousands of calories each day simply to maintain their bodyweight and fuel their training and game sessions. However, after their competitive careers ended they weren't nearly as active and thus didn't burn as many calories as they did when they were training and competing, with the result that a good many of them are now very fat. That doesn't mean that playing hockey will make you fat—and neither will bodybuilding training. As long as you match your calorie consumption to your energy expenditure, you needn't worry about your muscles "turning to" fat.

Train hard to stimulate a strength increase, allow enough time to recover and adapt, eat properly—and practice your skill set for the game of golf as often as possible. That's the most rational approach to improving your golf game.

SOURCES

BOOKS

Hatfield, Fred, *Bodybuilding: A Scientific Approach*. Chicago: Contemporary Books, 1988.

Lamb, David R. *Physiology of Exercise: Responses and Adaptations*. New York: MacMillan, 1984.

McArdle, William D., Frank I. Katch, and Victor L. Katch. *Exercise Physiology*. Philadelphia: Lea and Febiger, 1986.

Selye, Hans. *Stress Without Distress*. New York: New American Library, 1974.

Little, John, and Peter Sisco. *The Golfer's Two-Minute Workout*. New York: McGraw Hill, 1998.

JOURNALS

Berger, R. A. "Comparison of the effect of various weight training loads on strength." *Research Quarterly* 36:141–146, 1963.

Herbert, R. D., and M. Gabriel. "Effects of stretching before and after exercising on muscle soreness and risk of injury: systematic review." *British Medical Journal* 325:468–470, 2002.

Pope, R. P., R. D. Herbert, J. D. Kirwan, et al. "A randomized trial of preexercise stretching for prevention of lower-limb injury." *Medicine & Science in Sports & Exercise* 32:271–7, 2002.

Shrier, I. "Stretching before exercise does not reduce the risk of local muscle injury: a critical review of the clinical and basic science literature." *Clinical Journal of Sports Medicine* 9:221–227, 1999.

Thibault, M. C., et al. "Inheritance of human muscle enzyme adaptation to isokinetic strength training." *Human Heredity* 36 (6):341–7, 1986.

ONLINE REFERENCES

http://saveyourself.ca/articles/stretching.php
http://saveyourself.ca/bibliography.php?her00
http://news.bbc.co.uk/2/hi/health/2221716.stm
http://seriousstrength.com/flexibility.php
http://www.bmj.com/cgi/content/abstract/325/7362/468

ACKNOWLEDGMENTS

The author would like to thank both the Windermere Golf & Country Club and Muskoka Highlands (Muskoka, Ontario) for allowing us to photograph their beautiful courses. Also, the author would like to thank Jeremy Hymers for his participation in both the golf and exercise photo shoots. I would also like to acknowledge the hard work and contribution of two excellent trainers, particularly Cary Howe (who was extremely helpful during my two research projects at Nautilus North, and who is one of the best personal trainers on the planet) and Blair Wilson (who was the first to test the effects of hockey practice and competition on body composition and thus open a new window through which to view the training requirements of athletes during the competitive season). The understanding of the principles espoused in this book by the three individuals mentioned above have made the author's life much easier, as well as the lives of the thousands of clients they have trained throughout the years.

ABOUT THE AUTHOR

For over twenty years, John Little has worked alongside sports' greatest fitness authorities, athletes, champions, and innovators—from Steve "Hercules" Reeves, Jackie Chan, and Arnold Schwarzenegger, to six-time Mr. Olympia Dorian Yates and high-intensity training pioneer Mike Mentzer. In addition, Little and his wife, Terri, are the owners of Nautilus North Strength & Fitness Centre (www.nautilusnorth.com), which *Ironman* magazine lauded as "one of the leading fitness research centers in North America." Little is a regular columnist for *Ironman* and the innovator of three revolutionary training protocols (Max Contraction Training, Static Contraction Training, and Power Factor Training). His articles are published in every major fitness publication throughout the world, and he has written more than thirty books on bodybuilding, martial arts, history, and philosophy. Little's methods have been called "revolutionary" by the bodybuilding community.